D1581538

Educ Cen Library

Gynaecological Oncology for the MRCOG and Beyond

Published titles in the MRCOG and Beyond series

Antenatal Disorders for the MRCOG and Beyond
by Andrew Thomson and Ian Greer

Fetal Medicine for the MRCOG and Beyond
by Alan Cameron, Lena Macara, Janet Brennand and Peter Milton

Gynaecological and Obstetric Pathology for the MRCOG
by Harold Fox and C. Hilary Buckley, with a chapter on Cervical Cytology
by Dulcie V. Coleman

Intrapartum Care for the MRCOG and Beyond
by Thomas F. Baskett and Sabaratnam Arulkumaran,
with a chapter on Neonatal Resuscitation by John McIntyre
and a chapter on Perinatal Loss by Carolyn Basak

Management of Infertility for the MRCOG and Beyond
by Allan A. Templeton et al.

Menopause for the MRCOG and Beyond *by Margaret Rees*

Menstrual Problems for the MRCOG
by Mary Ann Lumsden, Jane Norman and Hilary Critchley

Neonatology for the MRCOG *by Peter Dear and Simon Newell*

Reproductive Endocrinology for the MRCOG and Beyond
edited by Adam Balen

The MRCOG: A Guide to the Examination *by Ian Johnson et al.*

Forthcoming titles in the series

Early Pregnancy Issues

Gynaecological Urology

Molecular Medicine

Gynaecological Oncology for the MRCOG and Beyond

Edited by David Luesley and Nigel Acheson

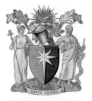

RCOG Press

Published by the **RCOG Press**
at the Royal College of Obstetricians and Gynaecologists
27 Sussex Place, Regent's Park, London NW1 4RG

www.rcog.org.uk

Registered charity no. 213280

First published 2004

ISBN 1-900364-85-9

Cover illustration: Mosaic and punctation

RCOG Editor: Jane Moody

Design/typesetting: Tony Crowley

Printed by Latimer Trend & Co. Ltd., Estover Road, Plymouth PL6 7PL

Acknowledgements
We would both wish to thank our contributors for their timely efforts, patience and persistence. We have at one time or another worked together as a team and we both hope this text reflects a team effort.

David Luesley
Nigel Acheson

Contents

About the authors

Nigel Acheson MD MRCOG
Consultant Gynaecological Oncologist
Birmingham Women's Healthcare NHS Trust,
City Hospital, Metchley Park Road, Edgebaston, Birmingham, B15 2TG, UK.

Yuk Ming Chan MRCOG
Medical Officer and Accredited Gynaecological Oncologist
Division of Gynaecological Oncology, Department of Obstetrics and Gynaecology,
Queen Mary Hospital, 102 Pokfulam Road, Hong Kong, China.

Quentin Davies MD FRCS(ED) MRCOG
Consultant in Gynaecological Oncology
Leicester Royal Infirmary, Leicester, LE1 5WW

Ian Etherington MD MRCOG
Consultant Obstetrician and Gynaecologist
Sandwell and West Birmingham NHS Trust,
City Hospital, Dudley Road, Birmingham, B13 9SG, UK.

Raji Ganesan
Consultant Pathologist and Honorary Senior Lecturer
First Floor Laboratories, Birmingham Women's Healthcare NHS Trust,
City Hospital, Metchley Park Road, Edgebaston, Birmingham, B15 2TG, UK.

Susan Houghton MRCOG
Consultant Obstetrician and Gynaecologist
Department of Obstetrics and Gynaecology, Good Hope Hospital NHS Trust,
Rectory Road, Sutton Coldfield, West Midlands B75 7RR, UK.

David Luesley MA MD FRCOG
Professor of Gynaecological Oncology
Birmingham Women's Healthcare NHS Trust,
City Hospital, Metchley Park Road, Edgebaston, Birmingham, B15 2TG, UK.

Chris Mann MD MRCOG
Consultant Gynaecological Oncologist/Senior Lecturer in Gynaecological Oncology
Department of Obstetrics and Gynaecology, Birmingham Women's Healthcare NHS
Trust, City Hospital, Metchley Park Road, Edgebaston, Birmingham, B15 2TG, UK.

Glyn Teale MRCP MRCOG FRANZCOG
Consultant Obstetrician and Gynaecologist
Goulburn Valley Health, Shepparton, Victoria 3630, Australia

Abbreviations

ACTION	Adjuvant Clinical Trial In Ovarian Neoplasm
AFP	alphafetoprotein
AIS	adenocarcinoma in situ
ASCO	American Society of Clinical Oncology
ASTEC	A Study in the Treatment of Endometrial Cancer
BEP	bleomycin [B], etoposide [E] and cisplatin [P] chemotherapy regimen
BIP	bleomycin [B], ifosfamide [I] and cisplatin [P] chemotherapy regimen
CAP	cisplatinum, adriamycin, cyclophosphamide chemotherapy regimen
CGIN	cervical glandular intraepithelial neoplasia
CIN	cervical intraepithelial neoplasia
CIS	carcinoma *in situ*
CMI	cell-mediated immunity
CK	cytokeratin
CT	computed tomography
CTCN	coagulative tumour cell necrosis
EMA-CO	etoposide [E], methotrexate [M], actinomycin D [A] cyclophosphamide [C], vincristine [O] chemotherapy regimen
ER	oestrogen receptor
FBC	full blood count
FIGO	International Federation of Gynecology and Obstetrics
GCDFP	gross cystic disease fluid protein
GOG	Gynaecological Oncology Group
GTD	gestational trophoblastic disease
GTT	gestational trophoblastic tumour
hCG	human chorionic gonadotrophin
HLA	human leucocyte antigen
HMFG	human milk fat globulin
HNPCC	hereditary non-polyposis colorectal cancer
HPV	human papillomavirus

HRT	hormone replacement therapy
HSIL	high-grade squamous intraepithelial lesions
ICON	International Collaboration on Ovarian Neoplasms
ISGP	International Society of Gynecological Pathologists
IVU	intravenous urogram
LFT	liver function tests
LLETZ	large loop excision of the transformation zone
LSIL	low-grade squamous intraepithelial lesions
MDA	minimum deviation adenocarcinoma
MPA	medroxyprogesterone acetate
MRI	magnetic resonance imaging
NHSCSP	National Health Service Cervical Screening Programme
NICE	National Institute for Clinical Excellence
PCR	polymerase chain reaction
POMB-ACE	cisplatin, vincristine, methotrexate and bleomycin; and actinomycin D, cyclophosphamide and etoposide chemotherapy regimen
PSTT	placental site trophoblastic tumour
PVB	cisplatin [P], vinblastine [V], bleomycin [B] chemotherapy regimen
SERM	selective oestrogen receptor modulator
STUMP	smooth muscle tumour of unknown malignant potential
TFT	thyroid function tests
TNM	tumour classification system based upon the state of the tumour, nodes and metastases
TVS	transvaginal scan
U&Es	urea and electrolytes
VAC	vincristine [V], actinomycin D [A]and cyclophosphamide [C] chemotherapy regimen
VAIN	vaginal intraepithelial neoplasia
VIN	vulval intraepithelial neoplasia
WHO	World Health Organization

Introduction

There has been considerable re-engineering of cancer services in the UK and elsewhere over the last decade. Formerly, obstetricians and gynaecologists were trained as and functioned as true generalists who might have to perform a radical hysterectomy for carcinoma of the cervix and yet also provide maternity, fertility and urological services. The emerging subspecialties and the vastly increased amount of information now make this approach less attractive to patients and specialists alike. However, just as there are subspecialists, the reorganisation of services also recognises that those tasked with general or other specialist areas of service provision require a level of knowledge in oncology equal to, if not exceeding, the generalists of previous years. Gynaecological oncology is still very much a part of the MRCOG curriculum and while one might not expect a recently qualified MRCOG candidate to be able to perform radical surgery or manage the acute complications of non-surgical therapies, one would expect a solid basic knowledge and understanding of the subdiscipline. In the UK we are aspiring to provide a truly network-based system of care that should be inclusive and not the exclusive preserve of those solely trained as subspecialists. In order for patients to access the network quickly and efficiently there must be a high level of expertise maintained throughout the profession.

This book aims to provide the basic core knowledge to achieve the first step in gaining this expertise. Many will wish to develop their skills further and some may go on to provide a subspecialist service. The book has been written by a local team whose members have had almost 15 years' experience in training gynaecological cancer specialists and being trained. In addition, the authors all currently work in an environment where the network model is well advanced and the value of cross-network multidisciplinary working is well accepted.

The text does not aim to be comprehensive but to furnish the reader with the basic facts and an appreciation of how to approach the more common oncological problems.

David Luesley
Nigel Acheson
June 2003

1 Basic epidemiology

Introduction

In recent years there has been a focus on the epidemiology of malignant disease, revealing links such as that between cigarette smoking and lung cancer. Epidemiologists are now investigating characteristics of individuals (e.g. genetic factors) or their environment (e.g. infections and drugs) that may play a part in the development of various cancers.

Information from epidemiological studies is helping to clarify the aetiology of gynaecological cancers. For example, the recognition of preinvasive changes in the genital tract has led to the establishment of cervical screening programmes and of the link with human papillomavirus (HPV), as well as an understanding of the role of oestrogen in the development of endometrial cancer. This in turn is helping to plan future prevention and treatment strategies. Table 1.1 shows the incidence, mortality and five-year survival rates for various cancers.

Cervical cancer

Cervical cancer is a potentially preventable disease yet it is the second most common cancer in women worldwide. In the UK, cervical cancer is the third most common malignancy to affect the genital tract, after ovarian and endometrial cancer.

The incidence of the disease in the UK has started to change. From 1971 to the mid-1980s, the incidence of cervical cancer remained fairly constant at 14–16/100000 but, since 1990, the incidence has fallen to just

Table 1.1 Tumour incidence, mortality and five-year survival, UK

Tumour site	New cases 1997 (n)	Deaths 1999 (n)	Overall five-year survival 1986–1990 (%)
Cervix	3240	1265	61
Uterus	4850	1395	70
Ovary	6820	4476	28

over 10/100000. By 1997, a total of 3240 cases had been registered, which represents 3% of all cancers in women (excluding non-melanoma skin cancer). However, the age-specific incidence has altered differently in the various age groups, with peak incidences of the disease occurring at 35–39 years and 75–79 years and significant decreases at 30–34 years and 70–74 years. These age-specific incidence trends suggest a birth–cohort effect, with peaks in risk for women born at the end of the 19th century, in the mid-1920s and after 1950. The latest figures from the National Health Service Cervical Screening Programme (NHSCSP) show that by 1996 the incidence had fallen to 8.9/100 000, representing an overall decrease in the incidence of cervical cancer of 42% over a six-year period.

The mortality associated with cervical cancer has fallen over the second half of the last century in the UK. From 1950 to 1987, the mortality rate decreased annually at a rate of 1.5%, from 11.2/100000 to 6.1/100000. The rate of decrease then trebled until 1997, by which time the mortality rate was 3.7/100 000, a total of 1150 deaths, which represented 2% of cancer deaths in women and 0.4% of all deaths in women. In a manner similar to that of incidence trends, the mortality trends also show a birth cohort effect. For example, the risk for women born in 1922 compared with the risk for those women born in 1957 is increased 1.5 times. This increased risk for women born after 1935 coincides with liberalised sexual behaviour associated with the 'swinging sixties'.

CERVICAL CANCER AND HUMAN PAPILLOMAVIRUS

The link between HPV and cervical cancer has been conclusively established. Of the 120 plus subtypes of HPV, around 20 have an association with the lower genital tract. Of these, the most important with respect to the risk of developing cervical cancer are HPV-16 and HPV-18.[1] See also Chapter 3 for a fuller discussion of HPV.

RISK FACTORS

Oncogenes
Normal cell regulation signals may be altered by oncogenes. Over-expression of certain oncogenes has been described in many cancers and some studies have linked this with the risk of progression from low- to high-grade cervical intraepithelial neoplasia (CIN).[2]

Genotype
The development of neoplasia in response to HPV infection is to a large extent determined by the host's response to that infection. A link has been reported between women who have the human leucocyte antigen (HLA) DQw3 genotype and cervical cancer.[3] It has also been reported that

women with cervical cancer who have the HLA B7 genotype have a poorer prognosis compared with other HLA types.[4] These associations probably reflect the different ways in which particular HLA molecules present HPV peptides to the immune system, with some HLA types being more efficient than others.

Smoking

There is strong epidemiological evidence linking smoking with CIN and cervical cancer.[5] The mechanism for this is unclear but it may be related to a direct mutagenic effect upon cervical squamous cells or to a resulting impaired immune response to HPV infection.[6] Products of smoking such as cotinine, nicotine, hydrocarbons and tars have been isolated in cervical mucus. However, virgins who smoke are not at increased risk of developing cervical cancer. So the presence of a chemical carcinogen alone is not sufficient. Another mechanism, which may explain the association, is the reduced numbers of antigen presenting Langerhans cells in cigarette smokers.[7] Langerhans cells are dendritic cells responsible for antigen presentation to the immune system. Studies have also found that cutting down or stopping smoking is associated with regression of low-grade CIN.[8]

Hormonal contraception

Women on the pill seem to have an increased incidence of cervical cancer[9] and the risk of developing glandular lesions appears even higher.[10] This risk is independent of the increased chance of contracting HPV if barrier contraception is not used. Why should this be the case? Eversion induced by oestrogen stimulates metaplasia, which could lead to an increased risk, and there may be a promotion of expression of viral proteins in women on the pill.

A full discussion of preinvasive disease of the cervix and screening as a preventive strategy is found in Chapter 3.

Dietary factors

Studies suggesting dietary associations are difficult to control for confounding variables. However there is some evidence for a protective effect of beta-carotene, vitamin C and folic acid.[11,12]

Endometrial cancer

Endometrial cancer is the second most common gynaecological cancer in the UK, principally affecting postmenopausal women. In the UK, there are approximately 5000 cases of endometrial cancer diagnosed each year, with around 1400 deaths from the disease each year. Only about 2–5% of cases occur before the age of 40 years. The incidence of endometrial cancer is low (less than two per 100000) in women under 40 years old but rises rapidly between the ages of 40 and 55 years, levelling off after the menopause at around 44 per 100000.

Most women with endometrial cancers develop abnormal vaginal bleeding as an early symptom and their tumours are diagnosed while confined to the uterus. Eight to ten percent of women with postmenopausal vaginal bleeding have cancer. Surgical excision by hysterectomy is often sufficient to treat the disease, but radiotherapy is used when the cancer is more advanced. Recent figures for England show that the age-standardised five-year survival rate is just over 70%. While around 90% of cases are diagnosed in women over the age of 50 years, younger women can develop the disease. In such cases, symptoms such as intermenstrual bleeding may occur and the diagnosis should be excluded in women with the risk factors cited below.

Some of the strongest epidemiological evidence in the field of gynaecological oncology links the effect of oestrogen upon the endometrium with the development of endometrial cancer.

RISK FACTORS

Obesity
In obese women, circulating oestrogen levels are raised by the conversion of androgens in peripheral fat. These androgens, androstenedione and testosterone, are produced by the adrenal glands.

Polycystic ovary syndrome
Women with polycystic ovary syndrome have an increased risk of endometrial cancer. The long, irregular menstrual cycles are associated with anovulation and unopposed oestrogen stimulation. This is explained by the fact that since the duration of the luteal phase is relatively constant, prolongation of the follicular phase results in the long cycles.

Parity
Nulliparous women are at increased risk of developing endometrial cancer. The protective effect of pregnancy appears to be greatest following the first pregnancy, with only modest decreases in risk seen with subsequent pregnancies.

Oral contraceptive pill
A protective effect of the oral contraceptive pill against the development of endometrial cancer is supported by robust epidemiological evidence. The protective effect increases with duration of use but appears to persist for 10–15 years after stopping the pill.

Unopposed oestrogen hormone replacement therapy
The risk of endometrial hyperplasia and neoplasia following the use of unopposed oestrogen in women with an intact uterus has been well known for over 20 years. A large review published by Grady et al. in 1995 assessed 30 studies with adequate controls and risk estimates.[13] The summary relative risk was 2.3 (range 2.1–2.5) for unopposed oestrogen, rising to 9.5 for ten or more years of use. The risk remained elevated at 2.3 five years after cessation of use.

The accepted practice of adding at least ten days of progestogen reduces the relative risk to between 1.0 and 1.8. The relative risk of endometrial cancer death is 2.7 for unopposed oestrogen.

Women with an intact uterus must not be given unopposed oestrogen hormone therapy.

Anti-oestrogens
Tamoxifen is a selective oestrogen receptor modulator (SERM). It is widely used in the treatment of breast cancer because it competes for oestrogen receptors in the breast. However, it stimulates ovarian oestrogen biosynthesis and elevates plasma oestrogen levels. This increases the risk of endometrial cancer. The relative risk for tamoxifen use of over five years has been estimated as 2.0. Newer SERMs have been developed in attempts to produce the ideal SERM, which would have no unwanted effects upon oestrogen receptors. One of these, raloxifene, has been shown to have anti-oestrogenic effects upon both the breast and endometrium. The risk of endometrial stimulation leading to endometrial cancer could therefore be abolished by using these newer SERMs that are currently under evaluation.[14]

Feminising ovarian tumours
Although rare, feminising ovarian tumours are a risk factor for the development of endometrial cancer. The tumour may be benign (thecoma) or malignant (granulosa cell tumour). Such a diagnosis should be borne in mind in women with evidence of oestrogenic endometrial stimulation that is otherwise unexplained.

Ovarian cancer

Ovarian cancer is the fifth most common cancer in women. In the UK, there are nearly 7000 cases of ovarian cancer diagnosed each year, with around 4500 deaths from the disease each year. It is the most common cause of gynaecological cancer death and affects approximately one in 70 women, with 50% of cases (49/100 000) occurring over the age of 65 years (Table 1.2).[15] This figure exceeds the number of women dying

Table 1.2   Five-year survival of ovarian cancer per FIGO stage

Stage	Five-year survival (%)
All	35–42
I	70–100
II	55–63
III	10–27
IV	3–15

from cervical and endometrial cancers combined. According to data from the International Federation of Gynecology and Obstetrics, five-year all-stage survival has increased from 27% in the early 1960s to 42% in the early 1990s. Unfortunately, although these data are encouraging, the silent nature of this disease results in 75% having extraovarian spread at the time of diagnosis (FIGO stage III or IV).

Epidemiological studies have shown that pregnancy, breastfeeding and oral contraceptive use appear to be protective against the development of ovarian cancer. These observations led to the incessant ovulation theory as a possible mechanism of oncogenesis. The basis of this theory is that the repeated mesothelial damage brought about by ovulation results in an increased possibility of a defect in the repair mechanism and eventually malignant transformation. Although superficially attractive, the reduction in incidence seen with just one pregnancy, a short exposure to combined oral contraception and the reduction in incidence occurring after hysterectomy with ovarian conservation have led many to doubt this hypothesis.

RISK FACTORS

Parity

Ovarian cancer is more common in nulliparous women and those of low parity. Initial cohort analyses in England and Wales, USA and Denmark suggested that increased parity was protective. Evidence from subsequent studies confirms that the reduction of ovarian cancer risk is around 10–16% for each pregnancy.[16] To a lesser degree, breastfeeding seems to further reduce the risk of developing ovarian cancer.

Genetic predisposition

Genetic predisposition to epithelial ovarian cancer occurs in up to 10% of patients with the disease, but only 7% of patients give a family history of ovarian cancer. A familial association in some patients with breast and ovarian cancers has been recognised for many years. BRCA 1 and BRCA 2 have been identified as tumour suppressor genes, with mutations being responsible for these familial cases. BRCA 1 is found on chromosome 17 and BRCA 2 on chromosome 13. Those with BRCA 1 mutations have a 40–60% lifetime risk of developing ovarian cancer, while for those with BRCA 2 mutations the risk is lower, at 10–20%. One of the two variants of hereditary non-polyposis colorectal cancer (HNPCC) has also been shown to have an association with ovarian cancer. Known as the Lynch type-II variant of HNPCC, it is associated with a 5–10% lifetime risk of developing ovarian cancer. In addition to the risk of ovarian cancer, women with this variant of HNPCC also have a 30% lifetime risk of developing endometrial cancer.[17]

Discovery of these gene mutations has led to attempts to screen families for the mutations. Currently over 100 mutations of BRCA 1 have been identified and detecting a mutation in the gene can therefore be difficult. Counselling of those considering such screening must address the difficult issue of managing those in whom a mutation is detected. In young women, future fertility is important and screening, together with estimation of serum CA125 levels and transvaginal ultrasound scanning (TVS), may be of benefit and is currently under investigation in a large national trial, UKCTOCS (the United Kingdom Collaborative Trial of Ovarian Cancer Screening). As previously mentioned, there is also evidence to suggest that the oral contraceptive pill may offer some protection to these patients.[18] Ultimately, however, prophylactic oophorectomy is likely to provide the greatest benefit. Because ovarian cancers in those with a genetic predisposition occur at an earlier age than sporadic cases, prophylactic surgery is recommended upon completion of a patient's family. It should be noted that in assessing families with a history suggestive of a genetic predisposition, the index case must be shown to carry a genetic mutation, and not to have been a sporadic case.

Oral contraceptive use

Epidemiological studies have shown a significant reduction in ovarian cancer risk in women who have used the combined oral contraceptive pill. With any use the risk of developing ovarian cancer may be reduced by 36%, with a reduction of up to 70% after six years.[18]

For women with a high risk of developing ovarian cancer (such as those with the BRCA 1 or BRCA 2 mutations), studies suggest that this risk can be reduced by 60% by using the combined oral contraceptive pill.[19] There is now a suggestion that the progestogen-only pill may confer an even greater level of protection. The mechanism of action is still somewhat speculative, but progestogens may promote apoptosis in ovarian mesothelium.[20]

Infertility

The possibility of a link between ovulation and ovarian oncogenesis led to concerns that infertility treatments might increase the risk of developing ovarian cancer. An association with ovulation induction has been difficult to elucidate. Initial studies appeared to suggest an increased risk but more recent studies have not confirmed this. Instead, it seems possible that the slightly increased numbers of cancers observed could be due to the increased risk associated with nulliparity. Despite the lack of evidence, women seeking ovulation induction should be counselled with regard to this possible association.

Squamous vulval cancer

Like skin cancers elsewhere, 90% of vulval cancers are squamous in origin. The remainder include melanomas, adenocarcinomas and sarcomas. In the UK there are around 900 cases of squamous vulval cancer diagnosed each year, with around 300 deaths from the disease each year. In 1996, 340 deaths were accorded to vulval carcinoma. This results in a crude death rate of 1.29 per 100000. Apart from its rarity, it is a condition that largely affects the elderly: 80% of women with this condition are over 55 years of age. It is not therefore surprising that medical co-morbidity is high in the vulval cancer population. Such co-morbidity poses additional challenges for management and may often influence choices of treatment.

The aetiology is poorly understood, but it now seems likely that vulval cancer develops in more than one way. HPVs (HPV-16 in particular) have been implicated in the development of vulval intraepithelial neoplasia (VIN) and the subsequent progression to cancer. In addition, patients with maturation disorders, such as lichen sclerosus, have an association with invasive vulval carcinoma. Thus, it seems likely that a second mechanism is responsible for malignant transformation. See Chapter 13 for further information on vulval cancer.

RISK FACTORS

Squamous vulval intraepithelial neoplasia

VIN is an uncommon condition, and its true incidence is unknown. The incidence of the condition has been thought to be increasing, by up to three-fold.[21,22] Interestingly, the incidence of vulval cancer has remained unchanged. The change in incidence of VIN could be due to an increased awareness of the condition leading to increased detection rates. The increased incidence of VIN is in part due to an increase in the number of young women in whom there appears to be a close association with HPV infection. The link between HPV, cervical intraepithelial neoplasia (CIN) and cervical cancer is well known. The situation is not so clear in patients with HPV and VIN. The incidence of VIN is increasing, particularly in young women with evidence of HPV infection. The incidence of vulval cancer is not increasing and the majority of patients developing cancer at present are older women with VIN not associated with HPV. A small group of women will have several genital tract neoplasias present at the same time, e.g. VIN, CIN and vaginal intraepithelial neoplasia (VAIN). One study has suggested that such changes are found in up to 25% of patients with VIN.[23] These patients present a long-term challenge in managing premalignant changes throughout the genital tract.

Lichen sclerosus

This uncommon disease can affect men and women, with women affected almost six times more commonly than men. Postmenopausal women are the most common group to be affected, although premenopausal women and even young girls can develop the disease.

SUMMARY

Cervix
- Increased risk of developing cervical cancer with increasing number of partners.
- Causal link between HPV and cervical cancer.

Endometrium
- Increased risk with obesity, polycystic ovary syndrome, nulliparity, unopposed oestrogen hormone replacement therapy, tamoxifen, feminising ovarian tumours.
- Decreased risk with increasing parity, oral contraceptive use.

Ovary
- Decreased risk with parity, breastfeeding and oral contraceptive pill use.
- Increased risk with nulliparity (and possibly infertility), genetic predisposition.

Vulva
- Link with both HPV and maturation disorders.

Various aetiological factors have been suggested. Of these, only the link between autoimmune disorders and lichen sclerosus has been clearly demonstrated. One study found that 21.5% of female patients had a history of autoimmune disease, such as thyroid disease, pernicious anaemia and diabetes.[24]

Long-term follow-up is recommended for patients with lichen sclerosus. This is based on the risk of malignant transformation, which is thought to be as high as 5% in some series.[25]

References

1. Schoell WM, Janicek MF, Mirhashemi R. Epidemiology and biology of cervical cancer. *Semin Surg Oncol* 1999; **16**: 203–11.

2. Hayashi Y, Hachisuga T, Iwasaka T, Fukada K, Okuma Y, Yokoyama M, *et al*. Expression of ras oncogene produce and EGF receptor in cervical squamous cell carcinomas and its relationship to lymph node involvement. *Gynecol Oncol* 1991; **40**: 147–51.

3. Wank R, Thomssen C. High risk of squamous cell carcinoma of the cervix for women with HLA-DQw3. *Nature* 1991; **352**: 723–5.

4. Ellis JRM, Keating PJ, Baird J, Hounsell EF, Renouf DV, Rowe M, *et al*. The association of an HPV 16 oncogene variant with HLA-B7 has implications for vaccine design in cervical cancer. *Nat Med* 1995; **1**: 464–70.

5. Trevathan EP, Layde LA, Webster DW, Adams JB, Benigno BB, Ory H. Cigarette smoking and dysplasia and carcinoma-in-situ of the uterine cervix. *JAMA* 1983; **250**: 499–505.

6. Kjellberg L, Hallmans G, Ahren AM, Johansson R, Bergman F, Wadell G, *et al*. Smoking, diet, pregnancy and oral contraceptive use as risk factors for cervical intra-epithelial neoplasia in relation to human papilloma virus infection. *Br J Cancer* 2000; **82**: 1332–8.

7 Barton SE, Jenkins D, Cizick J, Maddox PH, Edwards R, Singer A. Effect of cigarette smoking on cervical epithelial immunity – a mechanism for neoplastic change. *Lancet* 1988; **ii**: 652–4.

8. Szarewski A, Jarvis MJ, Sasieni P, Anderson M, Edwards R, Steele SJ, *et al*. Effect of smoking cessation on cervical lesion size. *Lancet* 1996; **347**: 941–3.

9. Salazar EL, Sojo-Aranda I, Lopez R, Salcedo M. The evidence for an etiologic relationship between oral contraceptive use and dysplastic change in cervical tissue. *Gynecol Endocrinol* 2001; **15**: 23–8.

10. Chilvers C, Mant D, Pike MC. Cervical adenocarcinomas and oral contraceptives. *BMJ* 1987; **295**: 1446–7.

11. Butterworth CE, Hatch K, Macaluso M. Folate deficiency and cervical dysplasia. *JAMA* 1992; **267**: 528–33.

12. Schneider A, Shah K. The role of vitamins in the etiology of cervical neoplasia: An epidemiological review. *Arch Gynecol Obstet* 1989; **246**: 1–13.

13. Grady D, Gebretsadik T, Kerlikowske K, Ernster V, Petitti D. Hormone replacement therapy and endometrial cancer risk: a meta-analysis. *Obstet Gynecol* 1995; **85**: 304–13.

14. Dhingra K. Selective estrogen receptor modulation: the search for an ideal hormonal therapy for breast cancer. *Cancer Invest* 2001; **19**: 649–59.

15. Yancik R. Ovarian cancer. Age contrasts in incidence, histology, disease stage at diagnosis, and mortality. *Cancer* 1993; 71 **Suppl**: 517–23.

16. Banks E, Beral V, Reeves G. The epidemiology of epithelial ovarian cancer: a review. *Int J Gynecol Cancer* 1997; **7**: 425–38.

17. Brown GJ, St John DJ, Macrae FA, Aittomaki K. Cancer risk in young women at risk of hereditary nonpolyposis colorectal cancer: implications for gynecologic surveillance. *Gynecol Oncol* 2001; **80**: 346–9.

18. Hankinson SE, Colditz GA, Hunter DJ, Spencer TL, Rosner B, Stampfer MJ. A quantitative assessment of oral contraceptive use and risk of ovarian cancer. *Obstet Gynecol* 1992; **80**: 708–14.

19. Narod SA, Risch H, Moleshi R, Dorum A, Neuhausen S, Olsson H, *et al*. Oral contraceptives and the risk of hereditary ovarian cancer. *N Engl J Med* 1998; **339**: 424–8.

20. Yu S, Lee M, Shin S, Park J. Apoptosis induced by progesterone in human ovarian cancer cell line SNU-840. *J Cell Biochem* 2001; **82**: 445–51.

21. Iversen T, Tretli, S. Intra-epithelial and invasive squamous cell neoplasia of the vulva: trends in incidence, recurrence and survival rate in Norway. *Obstet Gynecol* 1998; **91**: 969–72.

22. Sturgeon SR, Brinton LA, Devesa SS, Kurman RJ. In situ and invasive vulvar cancer incidence trends (1973 to 1987). *Am J Obstet Gynecol* 1992; **166**: 1482–5.

23. Shafi MI, Luesley DM, Byrne P, Samra JS, Redman CW, Jordan JA, *et al*. Vulval intra-epithelial neoplasia: management and outcome. *Br J Obstet Gynaecol* 1989; **96**: 1339–44.

24. Rowell NR, Goodfield MJD. The connective tissue diseases. In: Champion RM, Burton JL, Burns DA, editors. *Textbook of Dermatology*. Vol. 2. 6th ed. Oxford: Blackwell Science; 1998. p. 2547–53.

25. Meyrick Thomas RH, Ridley CM, McGibbon DH, Black MM. Lichen sclerosus et atrophicus and autoimmunity: a study of 350 women. *Br J Dermatol* 1988; **118**: 41–6.

2 Basic pathology of gynaecological cancer

Introduction

The cellular pathologist plays an important role both as a diagnostician and in providing prognostic information by examination of specimens removed at surgery for gynaecological cancers. Ideally, the pathologist deals with every specimen in order to provide maximum information to the clinician and the patient. The pathologist is an essential member of the multidisciplinary tumour panel and, through discussion with other team members, helps in formulating important management decisions.

This section describes the salient features that would enable the gynaecologist to aid and understand the pathologist in this process.

Sending specimens to the laboratory

FIXATION

Most specimens are sent to the laboratory in fixative, most commonly 10% formalin (4% formaldehyde) solution. Fixation serves to:

- harden tissue to allow sectioning
- preserve tissue by preventing autolysis
- inactivate infectious agents
- enhance avidity for dyes.

Since fixation is such an important process, the requesting clinician can assist the pathologist by sending the tissue in adequate fixative (10–15 times in volume) and by opening large specimens along anatomical planes: this allows penetration of fixative.

THE REQUEST FORM

This accompanies the specimen and should contain the following information:

- patient details, to prevent misidentification, which can lead to serious errors

- clinician details, with contact information
- date and time of procedure
- clinical history, which should include
  - the purpose of surgery
  - history of prior known disease
  - history of current disease and treatment
  - an indication of urgency of diagnosis
  - menstrual history
  - smear history
  - any other relevant details.

FROZEN SECTIONS

Frozen sections are a suboptimal but rapid method of solidifying small pieces of tissue in order to make tissue sections for microscopic examination. The information from a frozen section is limited by sampling (only small amounts of tissue can be studied), lack of special studies and interpretive limitations. In gynaecological pathology, the scope of frozen sections is limited.

- In ovarian borderline tumours, it must be understood that invasion not diagnosed on frozen section may be revealed on permanent sections.
- In mucinous tumours, malignancy may be missed because of the heterogeneity of these tumours.
- Primary tumours cannot be differentiated from metastatic tumours.
- There may be a limited role for evaluating margins of a surface epithelial tumour of the vulva.

Gynaecological pathology

This is a brief elaboration of areas that are of interest in gynaecological pathology, especially in the area of oncology. The following discussion does not claim to be a substitute for any standard textbook of pathology.

Cervix

CERVICAL INTRAEPITHELIAL NEOPLASIA

CIN is the term used to describe proliferative intraepithelial squamous lesions that display abnormal maturation and cytonuclear atypia. Mitotic activity is often increased and abnormal mitotic forms may be seen. The most important feature is abnormal maturation and this is manifested by loss of polarity and cellular disorganisation. CIN has a three-tier grading system based on the level of involvement of the squamous epithelium by the abnormality. For further information on CIN, see Chapter 3.

GRADING SYSTEM FOR CIN
CIN1 Abnormality confined to basal third of epithelium
CIN2 Abnormality up to lower two-thirds of epithelium
CIN3 Abnormality involving superficial third of epithelium

Immature metaplasia and atrophy are benign lesions that are commonly difficult to differentiate from CIN.

INVASIVE SQUAMOUS CARCINOMA

The classification of invasive cancers is based on the most predominant cellular type. They are classified into large-cell keratinising and non-keratinising. A further group is small-cell non-keratinising, which some data suggest has a worse outcome than the other squamous variants. Histological grade does not appear to have a major influence on outcome. Depth of invasion and the presence of lymph node metastases appear to be the most important histological predictors of outcome. Invasion to a depth of less than 5 mm (with a maximal lateral diameter of 7 mm) is defined within the substage Ia.

FIGO STAGE 1A CARCINOMAS
- Also known as microinvasive carcinoma
- Maximum size: 5 mm deep and 7 mm in horizontal dimension
- Vascular space involvement does not affect staging
  - 1A1: maximum depth of stromal invasion – 3 mm
  - 1A2: maximum depth of stromal invasion – 5 mm
- Verrucous carcinoma is a well-differentiated squamous carcinoma with an extremely low risk of nodal metastasis.

CERVICAL GLANDULAR INTRAEPITHELIAL NEOPLASIA

Cervical glandular intraepithelial neoplasia (CGIN) is best divided into a two-tier grading system: high-grade CGIN, a relatively robust histopathological diagnosis with good inter-observer correlation, and low-grade CGIN, which may be under-reported (Table 2.1).

Distinguishing high-grade CGIN from microinvasive carcinoma is difficult and features that raise the possibility of invasion are: back-to-back arrangement of glands with little stroma; cribriform gland pattern; desmoplastic stromal response; and increased cytoplasmic eosinophilia.

Table 2.1 Features of high-grade cervical glandular intraepithelial neoplasia

Architectural	Cytological
Gland crowding	Cellular stratification
Branching and budding	Loss of cytoplasmic mucin
Presence of intraluminal papillary projections	Nuclear enlargement Loss of polarity Increased mitotic activity

INVASIVE ADENOCARCINOMA

Unlike its squamous counterpart, there is no clearly defined or universally accepted microinvasion category. The outcome in these cancers depends upon size, stage and grade. There are several different subtypes. These include mucinous, endometrioid, serous, mesonephric and clear cell. There is also an intestinal type of mucinous tumour. There may be difficulties in differentiating an endometrioid variant from a uterine primary.

Minimum deviation adenocarcinomas (adenoma malignum)

Minimum deviation adenocarcinoma (MDA) is an extremely well differentiated variant of endocervical adenocarcinoma with the following features:

- little or no cytological atypia
- little mitotic activity
- presence of glands deep within the cervical stroma beyond the normal crypt field
- sometimes vascular and perineural invasion
- a known association with ovarian sex cord stromal tumour with annular tubules (in Peutz–Jeghers syndrome) and mucinous neoplasms.

Other variants of endocervical adenocarcinoma include:

- villoglandular carcinoma, which occurs in young women. It is well differentiated, often only superficially invasive, and has a better prognosis than other forms of endocervical adenocarcinomas.
- serous papillary carcinoma, which must be differentiated from villoglandular carcinoma as it has poorer outcome.
- clear cell carcinoma
- mesonephric adenocarcinoma, which is an extremely rare neoplasm that arises from the mesonephric or wolffian remnants.

Histological mimics of cervical glandular intraepithelial neoplasia and endocervical adenocarcinoma are:

- endometriosis
- tuboendometrioid metaplasia
- microglandular adenosis
- hyperplasia of mesonephric remnants
- tunnel clusters
- diffuse laminar endocervical hyperplasia
- Arias-Stella reaction involving endocervical glands.

ADENOSQUAMOUS CARCINOMA

This variant appears more frequently in younger women. No data as yet support the concept of a poorer outcome, although anecdotal information suggests that this may be the case. They contain malignant squamous and glandular cells and it may also be possible to identify adjacent CIN and CGIN.

Endometrium

ENDOMETRIAL CARCINOMA

Carcinoma of the endometrium has increased in frequency compared with carcinoma of cervix. In the USA, it is now the most common gynaecological cancer. The most common histological pattern resembles that of the proliferative endometrium and is labelled endometrioid adenocarcinoma. Other important histological patterns to recognise are detailed in Table 2.2.

Table 2.2 Histological patterns of endometrial carcinoma		
Pattern of carcinoma	Prognosis	Comment
Villoglandular	Same as typical endometrioid carcinoma	Should not be confused with serous carcinoma
Secretory	Uncommon variant resembling early or mid-secretory endometrium	Associated with a good prognosis
Serous	Poor	Frequent deep myometrial invasion and peritoneal implantation
Clear cell	Poor	

ENDOMETRIAL HYPERPLASIA

Hyperplasia of the endometrium is characterised by an increase in glandular tissue relative to stroma, with concomitant architectural and sometimes cytological abnormalities. The International Society of Gynecological Pathologists (ISGP) and World Health Organization (WHO) have proposed a classification system in which architectural and cytological features are independently evaluated (Table 2.3).

Complex hyperplasia with atypia is difficult to separate from well-differentiated endometrial carcinoma. Helpful histological features include a complex cribriform pattern; intraglandular bridging and polymorphs; abnormal mitotic activity; fibroblastic stromal response.

RELATIONSHIP OF HYPERPLASIA TO CARCINOMA

- Malignant progression
  Atypical hyperplasia has shown progression rates of 30% to cancer, while hyperplasia without atypia has negligible progression rates.
- Morphology
  Atypical hyperplasia has a cytomorphology similar to well-differentiated carcinoma.
- Morphometry
  Various morphometric techniques (nuclear area, nuclear perimeter, volume percentage of epithelium of glands etc.) have shown that atypical hyperplasias are closer to carcinoma, while hyperplasia without atypia is closer to normal proliferative endometrium.
- Progesterone receptors
  Endometrial hyperplasia without atypia has a high level of progesterone receptors, while in atypical hyperplasias levels are lower than normal endometrium but higher than endometrial carcinomas.
- Clonal analysis with polymerase chain reaction (PCR)
  This technique has shown that both carcinomas and atypical hyperplasias are monoclonal lesions.
- Microsatellite instability has been demonstrated in atypical hyperplasias but not in hyperplasia without atypia.
- Plotting the microsatellite alterations in an endometrium that contains carcinoma and atypical hyperplasia has shown an evolution in microsatellite instability with retention of altered microsatellites seen in atypical areas.
- Some endometrial tumours have a stromal component (Table 2.4).

Table 2.3 World Health Organization (WHO) classification of hyperplasia of the endometrium

Pattern	Cytological atypia	WHO	Simplified WHO
Rounded glands with regular outlines	None	Simple hyperplasia	Endometrial hyperplasia
Closely packed glands with irregular outlines	None	Complex hyperplasia	Endometrial hyperplasia
Rounded glands with regular outlines	Focal	Simple hyperplasia with atypia	Atypical endometrial hyperplasia
Closely packed glands with irregular outlines	Multifocal or diffuse	Complex hyperplasia with atypia[a]	Atypical endometrial hyperplasia

[a] This pattern has about a 25% risk of progressing to carcinoma

Müllerian adenomyomas

- Adenomyoma of endocervical type
- Typical adenomyomas of endometrioid type
- Atypical polypoid adenomyoma
  - typically solitary, well circumscribed, polypoid lesions of reproductive age group women
  - endometrioid glands with varying degrees of architectural and cytological atypia are separated by myofibromatous stroma
  - may recur in up to 45% of patients.

Smooth muscle tumours of the uterus

The most common tumour of the smooth muscle in the uterus is the benign leiomyoma. Several variants have been described. Smooth muscle tumours of the uterus also include smooth muscle tumour of unknown malignant potential (STUMP) and leiomyosarcoma. The terminology surrounding these various tumours is shown in Table 2.5.

Ovary

OVARIAN TUMOURS

There are three main groups of primary ovarian tumours: epithelial tumours that are derived from müllerian epithelium; sex cord or stromal

Table 2.4   Endometrial tumours with a stromal component

				Carcinosarcoma	
Component	Endometrial stromal nodule	Endometrial stromal sarcoma	Adenosarcoma	Homologous	Heterologous
No epithelial	+	+	–	–	–
Epithelial – benign	–	–	+	–	–
Epithelial – malignant	–	–	–	+	+
Benign stromal	+	+ (invasive margin)	–	–	–
Malignant stromal	–	+ (invasive margin)	+	+	+ Containing cell types not normally seen in uterus

tumours, derived from the ovarian stroma, sex cord derivatives or both; and germ cell tumours, which originate from the ovarian germ cells. The most common malignant tumours are serous, mucinous and endometrioid adenocarcinomas. The following are the most common ovarian tumours:

- mature cystic teratoma (dermoid cyst of the ovary)
- serous cystadenoma
- mucinous cystadenoma
- serous carcinoma
- fibroma-thecoma
- borderline serous tumour
- endometrioid carcinoma
- borderline mucinous tumour
- mucinous carcinoma.

BORDERLINE SEROUS TUMOURS

These are characterised by complex branching of papillae either from the cyst lining or on the ovarian surface, cellular proliferation and stratification, variable nuclear atypia and mitotic activity, and clear demarcation from underlying stroma.

- Stromal microinvasion
  Focus or foci of destructive stromal invasion measuring less than 3 mm.

Table 2.5   Smooth muscle tumours of the uterus

Name	Features	Comment
Cellular and highly cellular leiomyoma	Cytologically bland Mitotic activity < 5 MFs/10 HPF	Benign
Leiomyoma with bizarre nuclei	Variable numbers of cytologically bizarre nuclei No CTCN Mitoses < 10 MFs/10 HPF	Benign
Mitotically active leiomyoma	5–15 MFs/10 HPF Commonly submucosal, typically secretory phase due to mitogenic effect of progestins May be associated with use of GnRH agonists	Benign
Leiomyosarcoma	CTCN, diffuse moderate to marked cytological atypia, usually high mitotic rate	Malignant
Myxoid smooth muscle tumour	Myxoid background Difficult to evaluate because of low mitotic activity and focal atypia	Difficult to predict, extensive sampling advised
Atypical leiomyoma	Diffuse significant atypia < 10 MFs/10 HPF No CTCN With higher mitotic activity	Low risk of recurrence, experience limited
Smooth muscle tumour of low malignant potential	CTCN present, no more than mild atypia, less than 10 MFs/10 HPF	Controversial category
STUMP	Other combination of features of concern falling short of leiomyosarcoma	

CTCN = coagulative tumour cell necrosis; HPF = high-power field; MFs = mitotic figures; STUMP = smooth muscle tumour of unknown malignant potential

In the absence of extra-ovarian disease, this does not alter the prognosis.

- Implants
  Deposits of tumour in peritoneum or omentum, seen in 15–30% of borderline serous tumours (Table 2.6).

MICROPAPILLARY SEROUS CARCINOMA

A histological variant of borderline serous tumour characterised by long thin papillae is seen arising directly from a large papilla. The usual

Table 2.6   Implants

Type of implant	Appearance	Implication
Non-invasive	Surface growth only	No prognostic significance
Desmoplastic	Desmoplastic response in underlying stroma, no invasion.	No prognostic significance
Invasive	Invasion of underlying tissue	Poorer outcome

hierarchical pattern in conventional serous tumours is not seen. When florid, it is believed to indicate a prognosis closer to a serous carcinoma even in the absence of stromal invasion.

PSEUDOMYXOMA PERITONEI

This is a condition in which the peritoneal cavity is filled with paucicellular pools of mucin. On microscopy, the cellular component often has a bland morphology. The currently favoured opinion is that the primary tumour in these cases is in the appendix and the ovarian neoplasm is a secondary site.

CLEAR CELL CARCINOMA

This pattern of tumour indicates a poorer prognosis and a poorer response to platinum-based chemotherapy than other morphological types of ovarian cancer.

SEX CORD TUMOUR WITH ANNULAR TUBULES

Up to one-third of women with these tumours have Peutz–Jeghers syndrome.

GRADING SYSTEM FOR VIN

VIN1 Abnormalities confined to basal layers (lower one-third)
VIN2 Dysplastic keratinocytes confined to lower two-thirds
VIN3 Abnormal cells occupy full thickness of the epithelium

PATTERNS OF VIN

Warty Presence of multinucleate cells and koilocytes indicative of human papillomavirus
Basaloid Smaller, more compact. basaloid cells with less pleomorphism and fewer atypical mitoses
Differentiated Abnormal cells confined to the basal and parabasal layers with keratin pearl formation

---

Vulva

VULVAL INTRAEPITHELIAL NEOPLASIA

The term VIN encompasses a spectrum of intraepidermal pathology of the vulval skin or mucosa, ranging from mild atypia to severe abnormalities amounting to carcinoma *in situ*.

SQUAMOUS CELL CARCINOMA

- Invasive tumour showing squamous differentiation
- Superficially invasive squamous carcinoma is a term used when the depth of invasion is $\leq$ 1 mm.
- Depth of invasion differs from tumour thickness.
- Depth of invasion: from the epithelial stromal junction of the most superficial adjacent normal dermal papilla to the deepest invasive tumour
- Tumour thickness: surface (if ulcerated) or granular layer of overlying keratinised surface to the deepest point of invasion.

VERRUCOUS CARCINOMA

This is a well-differentiated and biologically low-grade neoplasm. To fit into this category, strict histological criteria must be fulfilled. These include pushing borders, no frank destructive invasion and large keratinocytes with pale eosinophilic cytoplasm and sparse mitotic activity.

EXTRAMAMMARY PAGET'S DISEASE

The vulva is one of the most commonly involved sites. The origin of this neoplasm is unclear. Histological features are as follows:

- clonal nests or single pale cells in the epidermis
- rarely, invasive elements are seen
- mucin stains positive
- carcinoembryonic antigen (CEA), epithelial membrane antigen (EMA), gross cystic disease fluid protein-15 (GCDFP-15), CAM.5.2 all positive
- S100 negative: aids differentiating from melanoma.

MERKEL CELL CARCINOMA

Merkel cell carcinoma is a primary neuroendocrine carcinoma of the skin, predominantly occurring in the dermis. The lesion may appear as trabeculae or solid sheets of cells with scanty cytoplasm. The nuclei are hyperchromatic with inconspicuous nucleoli and overall the tumours show a high mitotic and apoptotic activity. They stain positive for neuroendocrine markers and 'dot-like' cytoplasmic positivity is seen with CAM.5.2 and cytokeratin 20 (CK20).

MELANOMA

- Melanoma accounts for about 9% of all malignant vulval tumours.
- Clark's levels of invasion can be applied to vulval melanomas.
- Breslow's thickness (in mm) measures the thickness of a melanoma.
- Immunohistochemically melanomas are positive for S100, HMB45 and Melan A.
- Poorer outcome is indicated by:
  - ○ Breslow's thickness greater than 0.76 mm
  - ○ Clark's level greater than II
  - ○ vascular involvement.

PERITONEAL PATHOLOGY

Mesothelial lesions

- Mesothelial hyperplasia
- Multicystic mesothelioma
  - ○ occurs predominantly in women of reproductive age
  - ○ involves the pelvic peritoneum
  - ○ may recur after surgical removal
- Well-differentiated papillary mesothelioma
  - ○ well-developed coarse papillae are seen
  - ○ clinical behaviour is usually prolonged and largely benign
- Malignant mesothelioma
  - ○ invasive tumour with poor prognosis.

Lesions of the secondary müllerian system

- Serous lesions
  - ○ endosalpingiosis
  - ○ peritoneal serous borderline tumours
  - ○ serous psammocarcinoma
  - ○ peritoneal serous carcinoma
- Mucinous lesions
  - ○ endocervicosis
  - ○ pseudomyxoma-like lesions with no appendiceal or ovarian abnormality
- Transitional lesions
  - ○ Walthard nests
  - ○ transitional cell neoplasms
- Ectopic decidua
- Diffuse peritoneal leiomyomatosis.

Table 2.7   Commonly used stains and their possible applications

Stain	Components stained	Comments
Periodic acid – Schiff stain (PAS)	Glycogen, neutral mucin	Highlights glycogen and mucin in cells
PAS with diastase digestion	Mucin	Glycogen is digested by diastase and therefore not stained
Alcian blue	Acid mucins	Can identify intestinal type mucin
Ziehl–Nielsen stain	Mycobacteria	To identify tuberculosis bacillus
Toluidine blue	Mast cells	

Special studies in pathology

The haematoxylin and eosin stain is the basic stain used primarily on every specimen by a pathologist. Familiarity with the special studies available is important for the clinician because the initial handling of the specimen may limit the types of studies that can be performed.

HISTOCHEMISTRY

All histochemical stains can be performed on formalin-based tissue. Table 2.7 shows the commonly used stains and their possible applications.

Table 2.8   Commonly used antibodies and their significance

Antibody	Tissue identified
Cytokeratin	Epithelial
S100	Neural, melanocytic
HMB45	Melanocytic
Vimentin	Mesenchymal
Inhibin	Sex cord elements
CA125	Mesothelial/müllerian
Leucocyte common antigen	Leucocytes
CD10	Endometrial stroma
Human chorionic gonadotrophin	Trophoblast
Human placental lactogen	Trophoblast
Placental alkaline phosphatase	Germ cell elements
Alphafetoprotein	Yolk sac elements
Smooth muscle antigen, desmin	Smooth muscle
Chromogranin	Neuroendocrine
Thyroglobulin	Thyroid

IMMUNOHISTOCHEMISTRY AS A DIAGNOSTIC TOOL

Immunohistochemistry or immunocytochemistry is a diagnostic tool used by cellular pathologists for accumulating evidence for or against a diagnostic possibility after the conventional stains have generated a differential diagnosis. This technique localises target antigens on cells with the help of antigen-specific antibodies (primary antibodies) applied to formalin-fixed, paraffin-embedded tissue sections. A secondary antibody-based reagent is then used to colour the target molecule at the specific interaction site. The specificity and sensitivity of the primary antibody, the presence of the antibody at the specific site and the perfection of techniques of antigen retrieval are important in interpretation of the results. Commonly used antibodies and their significance are shown in Table 2.8.

The major role of immunohistochemistry in diagnostic gynaecological pathology is in differentiating between primary and metastatic carcinoma of the ovary.

DIFFERENTIATING BETWEEN PRIMARY AND METASTATIC OVARIAN CANCER

Metastatic carcinomas to the ovary account for up to 7% of all ovarian neoplasms. Primary endometrioid carcinoma is closely mimicked by a metastatic colonic carcinoma. Differential staining with cytokeratin 7 (CK7) and CK20 can be used to separate these histologically similar entities (Table 2.9).

Obviously this staining pattern is not of use when evaluating the possibility of a metastatic breast carcinoma. Here a differential staining pattern with GCDFP-15 and oestrogen receptor (ER) is helpful (Table 2.10).

EVALUATION OF METASTATIC CARCINOMA

- Morphology
- Clinical history

Table 2.9	Differential staining to separate histologically similar entities	
CK20	CK7 positive	CK 7 negative
Positive	Urothelial carcinomas Pancreaticobilary carcinomas Mucinous ovarian neoplasms	Colorectal carcinomas
Negative	Breast carcinoma Non-mucinous ovarian carcinomas	Hepatocellular carcinomas Renal cell carcinomas
CK = cytokeratin		

- Operative findings – extra-ovarian tumour
- Histology – bilaterality, surface tumour, multinodularity, vascular invasion
- Clinical relevance of determining primary site
- Immunohistochemical panel – limiting panel to most powerful markers.

EXTRAMAMMARY PAGET'S DISEASE

Paget's disease versus superficially spreading melanoma (Table 2.11).

EVALUATING SPINDLE TUMOURS OF THE MYOMETRIUM

Endometrial stromal versus smooth muscle tumours (Table 2.12).

GLANDULAR LESIONS OF CERVIX

These immunohistochemical stains have yet to be approved for routine clinical applicability (Table 2.13).

PERITONEAL MESOTHELIOMA VERSUS SEROUS CARCINOMA IN THE PERITONEUM

These are difficult to distinguish histologically and, when there is diffuse involvement, immunohistochemistry can be of considerable ancillary value. In the differentiation between papillary serous carcinoma of the peritoneum and serous carcinoma of the ovary, immunohistochemical studies are of limited value as they have a similar phenotype.

Table 2.10   Evaluation of metastatic breast carcinoma

	CK7	CK20	GCDFP-15	ER
Breast	+	–	+	+/–
Ovarian non-mucinous primary	+	–	–	–/+
CK= cytokeratin; ER = oestrogen receptor; GCDFP = gross cystic disease fluid protein				

Table 2.11   Paget's disease versus superficially spreading melanoma

	S100	HMB45	CAM5.2	EMA
Paget's disease	–	–	+	+
Superficial spreading melanoma	+	+	–	–
EMA = epithelial membrane antigen				

Table 2.12 Endometrial stromal versus smooth muscle tumours

	CD10	CD34	SMA	Desmin	h-caldesmin
Endometrial stromal tumours	+	–	–	+ Focal	–
Smooth muscle tumours	–	+/–	+	+ Diffuse	+
SMA = smooth muscle antigen					

For the best diagnostic discriminants between epithelial mesotheliomas and serous carcinomas (note that serum CA125 has no diagnostic utility in this differential) see Table 2.14.

PROGNOSTIC VALUE OF IMMUNOHISTOCHEMICAL MARKERS

Cancer prognosis has always been based on histological typing and grading, imaging findings and clinical stage of the patients. While this is valid in population or group-based studies, it is of little direct relevance to the individual patient or tumour. Immunohistochemistry is now being used both at research and practice levels to identify subsets of patients who will be likely to benefit from additional therapy. Not all the methods listed below are in use for gynaecological tumours, but the list provides some indication of what lies ahead in the field of gynaecological oncology.

Tumour microstaging

The following will help to accurately stage tumours by detecting micrometastases or vascular invasion, thus aiding appropriate treatment:

- detection of microinvasion by use of quantitative and qualitative assessment of immunohistochemistry for basement membranes
- use of vascular markers (factor VIII-related protein, CD31, CD34) to detect vascular space involvement

Table 2.13 Glandular lesions of the cervix

	CEA	HMFG1	EMA	CD44v5
Normal epithelium	+/–ve/luminal+ve	+/–ve/luminal+ve	–ve/basolateral+ve	+ve
CGIN	cytoplasmic+ve	cytoplasmic+ve	+ Diffuse	–ve
CGIN = cervical glandular intraepithelial neoplasia; CEA = carcinoembryonic antigen; EMA = epithelial membrane antigen; HMFG1 = human milk fat globulin 1				

Table 2.14 Best diagnostic discriminants between epithelial mesothelioma and serous carcinoma

	Thrombomodulin	Calretinin	Keratin 5/6	Ber-Ep4	B72.3	CA125
Mesothelioma	+	+	+	–	–	+
Serous carcinoma	–	–	–	+	+	+

- detection of micrometastasis to lymph nodes and bone marrow by using immuno stains for relevant epithelial markers.

Markers to predict response to therapy

Oestrogen and progesterone receptors in breast cancer provide information for prognostication, as well as helping to inform decisions regarding hormonal manipulation of the tumour. Steroid-regulated proteins cathepsin D and pS2 serve as post-receptor markers for a functional oestrogen receptor pathway.

C-erbB-2 gene alterations have been reported in many tumours. In breast cancer, c-erbB-2 positive tumours can be treated with the anti c-erbB-2 drug herceptin.

Androgen receptor estimation is performed in prostatic carcinomas.

Estimation of tumour cell proliferation to provide an estimate of the tumour growth fraction

- Ki67 antigen
- P27kip1 gene
- proliferating cell nuclear antigen.

Others

- tumour suppressor genes
- tumour angiogenesis
- anti-apoptosis genes
- DNA repair genes
- adhesion molecules.

MOLECULAR GENETIC PATHOLOGY

This incorporates many techniques in use for the investigation of genetic alterations in cells and organisms. The techniques include polymerase chain reaction (PCR), Southern blotting and *in situ* hybridisation. Molecular genetic pathology has application in three main areas:

- identification of inherited diseases
- detection of microorganisms
- cancer: identification of specific genetic alterations, identification of clonality and detection of minimal residual disease.

3 Preinvasive disease of the lower genital tract

Introduction

This chapter concentrates mainly on premalignancy of the cervix, as this is the most common of the preinvasive conditions and the only one that is screened for on a population basis. Most of the information about cervical premalignancy refers to squamous lesions, as these are by far the most frequent, but preinvasive disease of glandular tissue will also be considered, as will preinvasive conditions of the vagina and vulva.

Preinvasive disease and terminology

The concept of precancer of the cervix dates back to the end of the 19th century, when Sir John Williams described non-invasive tissue resembling malignancy adjacent to an area of microinvasive carcinoma in a hysterectomy specimen. The term carcinoma *in situ* (CIS) was introduced in the 1930s. Retrospective studies on archived histological material found CIS lesions in women who subsequently went on to develop cervical cancer and so the precursor nature of CIS to cervical cancer came to be established. Subsequent prospective studies have confirmed these findings.[1,2]

When the Papanicolaou smear was introduced in the 1940s and abnormalities investigated it became obvious that there were changes not amounting to CIS but still showing similar features. These lesser changes were initially referred to as 'dysplasia' but because it was an imprecise term covering a range of abnormalities from normal to CIS many other terms were also in use. This caused confusion in management: women with CIS were usually treated by hysterectomy – sometimes radical hysterectomy – whereas those with dysplasia were often disregarded. In the 1960s, Richart introduced the term CIN and divided it into grades 1, 2 and 3. Grades 1 and 2 corresponded to mild and moderate dysplasia, respectively, and grade 3 combined severe dysplasia and CIS into one category.[3] The definition implied a continuum of change and emphasised to clinicians the concept of a single disease entity which it was hoped would lead to more rational management. The concept of a continuum of change from CIN1 to cervical cancer has now been challenged. The process seems to be a series of discrete events starting off with HPV infection. Progression or regression depends on several factors. For practical purposes a two-stage grading is now used, with CIN1 becoming low-grade CIN, where there is a significant chance for regression, and CIN2 and CIN3 being grouped together as high-grade CIN. In North America and some European countries this grouping has been formalised as the Bethesda classification consisting of low-grade squamous intraepithelial lesions (LSIL) and high-grade squamous intraepithelial lesions (HSIL), equivalent to mild and moderate/severe dyskaryosis, respectively.

Cervical precancer has a long natural history, which is one of the reasons why it is amenable to screening. If a cancer is going to develop at all it will take several years to do so, even from a CIN3 lesion. It is unclear why some CIN3 lesions become invasive while others stay as intraepithelial disease and it is not known how many CIN3 lesions will become invasive, since prospective studies are unethical. However the best prospective data suggest that between 30–50% of women with CIN3 would develop invasive cancer if left alone.[2]

At the other end of the spectrum we know that a significant proportion of women with minor disease will regress to normal if left untreated. Up to 50% of women with minor cytological abnormalities will revert to normal if left alone.[4] On the other hand, you could look at the figures and say that women with mild dyskaryosis have a 16–47 times increased incidence of invasive disease compared with the general female population.[5]

Human papillomaviruses

HPVs are small DNA viruses, about 55 nm in diameter, consisting of a single double-stranded circular chromosome of around 8000 base pairs and a 72-sided icosahedral protein coat (Figure 3.1). The chromosome is divided into early (E) and late (L) regions. The early region codes for functional proteins while the late region codes for the protein coat of the virus.

THE MAIN GENE PRODUCTS

E6   Transforming protein that can bind to the $p53$ tumour suppressor

E7   Major transforming protein that binds the RB tumour suppressor

L1   Major capsid protein

L2   Minor capsid protein

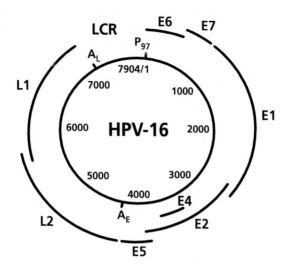

Figure 3.1 A schematic diagram of HPV

Many different types of HPV have been and continue to be identified. Currently over 100 types have been isolated. In addition to the different types there are subtypes (2–10% genomic variation compared with the prototype) and variants (< 2% genomic variation compared with prototype) to consider as well. Broadly speaking, they can be divided into mucosal and cutaneous types. Full virus particles are only expressed in the most superficial cells of the epithelium. As these cells are fully differentiated and cannot divide, the virus is unable to be grown in cell culture. DNA hybridisation techniques such as PCR or hybrid capture detects the presence of HPV. Currently, the only available commercial assay is Hybrid Capture® (Digene Corp.), which tests for a cocktail of HPV types depending on their oncogenic potential. Genital HPVs are divided in to higher-risk types (HPV-16, -18, -31, -33, -35, -45, -56 etc.) and lower-risk types (HPV-6, -11 etc.) depending on their association with malignancy. Indeed the WHO has formally classified HPV-16 and -18 as carcinogenic. Despite the last sentence, HPV should be regarded as an extremely common infection that rarely causes cancer. So how common is it? The figures vary depending on what test is used, with the highest figures being quoted where the testing has been by PCR. It has been estimated that 1% of American sexually active adults have visible genital warts and that 15–20% have subclinical infection detected by PCR.[6] This proportion rises to 30–40% if only young adults are considered. Some studies even found the prevalence to be > 80% but these were probably flawed due to contamination in early PCR work.[7] The figures quoted rely on testing for HPV DNA and so may not reliably assess previous infection. This can be done using serological tests seeking antibodies to capsid protein and it is likely that up to 75% of the population have been infected at some time in their lives with one or more genital HPV types.[8] These figures for prevalence of HPV and past exposure are vastly in excess of the number of cases of CIN, let alone cancer. So most infections, even with high-risk types, are transient and will be cleared in time by the host's immune responses. We know that the major immune response to HPV infection is cell mediated (CMI) because women with impaired CMI, such as transplant patients on immunosuppression or women with HIV infection, have an increased incidence of CIN and cervical cancer.[9] In contrast, women with impaired humoral immunity do not have an increased risk of HPV-associated problems.

Immortalisation and transformation

Most cells have a limited replication lifespan and can divide about 50–60 times. Infection with HPV prolongs this lifespan but eventually most of the cells stop proliferating and differentiate. Certain cell lines that have acquired genetic modifications escape differentiation and carry on dividing. This is called immortalisation. The E6 and E7 oncoproteins are necessary for this but vary in their ability to do so according to HPV type; E6 binds to the p53 cellular protein and E7 to the RB cellular protein, both of which are cell cycle regulators.[10,11] Interfering with the cell cycle allows DNA changes to accumulate, which may result in spontaneous transformation of the cell into a malignant cell line. This process may be accelerated by co-factors (see Chapter 1).

The NHS Cervical Screening Programme

A nationwide organised (as opposed to opportunistic) cervical screening programme was introduced with the computerised call-and-recall system in 1988. Prior to this, cervical screening varied in different areas of the country. The regions still have a degree of autonomy in planning their screening programme but there is now a National Co-ordinating Network to ensure the adoption of common standards and working practices. Regions are required to offer screening to women aged 20–64 years on a maximum five-yearly cycle. Most regions now screen three-yearly but the emphasis remains on coverage rather than frequency: it is far better to screen 100% of eligible women every five or even ten years than to screen 50% every two or three years. In other words, the women who are not screened are likely to be those at most risk of the disease. Nationwide coverage is now around 85%.[12]

Over 4.5 million smears are assessed annually in England to detect preinvasive changes and to help reduce the 3700 cases of invasive cervical cancer and the 1300 deaths each year. This is one of the major factors to consider when thinking about the frequency of screening events: if we screen every woman yearly she will have 45 smears taken in her life, compared with 15 if screening is three-yearly and nine if a five-year cycle is adopted. If we assumed maximum coverage for a five-yearly programme it has been estimated that 84% of cases of invasive cancer could be prevented; the figure for a three-yearly programme is 91% and the incremental gains become less and less thereafter with increasing screening frequency.[13] So in terms of cost–benefit there is little justification for reducing the screening interval. Because of the extremely low incidence of invasive cervical cancer in women below the age of 20 years and because of the high prevalence of HPV infection at this age, screening of women under 20 years is not justified. Of course some women under 20 years of age are screened, such as at a family planning clinic, but this screening is opportunistic and not part of the national programme. If teenagers were screened as well there would be a large increase in women with minor smear abnormalities requiring follow-up or investigation, the vast majority of whom would have transient HPV infection. Similarly, at the other end of the spectrum, provided that a woman has been adequately screened and provided she has not recently changed her partner, there is no justification for continuing with screening after the age of 65 years if the smear history is normal. Indeed, some authors have questioned the validity of screening such women beyond the age of 50 years.[14]

Cervical cytology is not a perfect test: data from the USA have estimated the specificity to be 98% and the sensitivity only 51%.[15]

RATES OF ABNORMALITY

About 92% of the smears taken are adequate for diagnosis and just under 10% of adequate smears are 'not normal'. Most smear abnormalities are at the minor end of the spectrum. Overall, 4.2% of smears are reported as borderline changes, 2.2% as mild dyskaryosis, 0.7% as moderate dyskaryosis and 0.6% as severe dyskaryosis.[16] Only 0.1% of smears are reported as suspected invasion or glandular neoplasia. In general the proportion of normal smears increases in older women but so does the proportion of abnormalities representing invasive cancer. Borderline changes and mild dyskaryosis are common in young women; the proportion of moderate dyskaryosis is highest for women aged 20–29 years and the proportion of severe dyskaryosis is highest in women aged 25–34 years.[16]

FURTHER INVESTIGATIONS

Women are referred for further investigation after one moderate or severe dyskaryosis smear result but if they have mild dyskaryosis the smear is repeated six months later and referral is then made if an abnormality persists. If a woman has a borderline smear it is repeated 6–12 months later and referral made on the basis of a persisting abnormality. This latter point presupposes that the cervix appears normal and that the woman has had negative smears to date.

By definition, a screening test is not diagnostic but merely identifies a subgroup of the reference population at increased risk of the disease where further tests should be carried out. In this case, the reference population being screened consists of healthy asymptomatic women. As the majority of women with 'at risk' tests will either have no risk or minimal risk of developing cancer, it is vitally important to carry out the process in a way which minimises the risk of them becoming patients with disease. The screening programme has the ability to generate much psychological morbidity, which may be compounded during the course of investigation.[17] Further investigation of smear abnormalities is by colposcopy.

THE COLPOSCOPIC EXAMINATION

A colposcope is a low-power binocular microscope, which illuminates the objective and allows for magnification from around four times to 25 times (Figure 3.2; plate 1). Most devices now incorporate a green filter, which enhances visualisation of structures containing red pigment (blood vessels). In the UK it is used to look for the source of the problem that has been identified by the abnormal smear. In other countries, which do not have organised cytological screening, it may be used as a primary tool. Indeed, the colposcope was invented long before Papanicolaou and Traut described cytological changes back in 1943: Hans Hinselmann invented the colposcope in the 1920s in Germany as a way of detecting early invasive cancers.

Before the actual examination, time should be taken to reassure the woman, gain her confidence and listen to her questions. A brief history is taken, noting particularly the date of her last period, whether or not she smokes and what contraception she is using. The vast majority of women can be reassured prior to the examination that they are extremely unlikely to have cancer: this is very important to emphasise.

The woman is examined on a purpose-built couch in a modified lithotomy position. Her cervix is exposed with a bivalve speculum and examined with the colposcope at low magnification (4–6x). A saline-soaked cottonwool ball is then applied to the cervix, which moistens the epithelium, allowing the underlying blood vessels to be examined. Higher magnification (preferably 16x or even 25x) is needed for this part of the examination. A green filter is a useful aid as it makes the capillaries stand out much more clearly. The various shapes of the capillaries can be studied and the intercapillary distances measured. Not all colposcopists use the saline technique but it can be particularly useful in difficult cases. Acetic acid (3% or 5%) is then applied using a cottonwool ball or by a spray.

In addition to its use in diagnosis, acetic acid has a mucolytic effect and so residual mucus can be cleared away prior to the examination. Areas of CIN will appear as varying degrees of whiteness. This is termed acetowhiteness (Figure 3.3; plate 1) in contrast to areas of hyperkeratosis or leukoplakia that appear white before application of acetic acid. The exact reason why CIN tissue turns white with acetic acid is not fully understood. The cytoplasm becomes dehydrated so in areas of abnormality where there is a high nuclear/cytoplasmic ratio in the cells the nuclei become crowded and the light from the colposcope is reflected back. Such areas will therefore appear white. However, not all areas of high nuclear density are abnormal and so not all acetowhiteness necessarily correlates with CIN: areas of regenerating epithelium, subclinical papillomavirus infection and immature metaplasia may also appear acetowhite. One of the challenges facing the colposcopist is to decide which areas of acetowhiteness truly represent premalignancy and to avoid treating benign conditions.

The classical vessel patterns of CIN are punctation and mosaicism (Figures 3.4 and 3.5; plates 2 and 3). Bizarrely shaped vessels suggest cancer. Another test used in the colposcopy clinic involves the application of Lugol's iodine solution to the cervix. Normal squamous epithelium contains glycogen and stains dark brown when Lugol's iodine is applied. Conversely, premalignant and malignant squamous tissue contains little or no glycogen and do not stain with iodine. This is Schiller's test: areas which are nonstaining with iodine are referred to as 'Schiller positive' and those which take up iodine as 'Schiller negative' (Figure 3.6; plate 3). The test may be used following acetic acid colposcopy.

The colposcopist uses many variables in forming a diagnosis of the underlying disease. What happens next depends on the diagnosis and the colposcopist. Everyone agrees that high-grade lesions (CIN2/3) should be treated but there is some debate about whether and when CIN1 should be treated. Some colposcopists will treat all lesions regardless of grade, whereas others will allow CIN1 lesions chance to regress. In considering which approach to adopt, the psychological impact of management policies on women should be considered: it is important that a woman is not labelled as having a sexually transmitted precancerous condition when she may only have a transient viral infection. If it is decided that treatment is needed there are a variety of options. Broadly speaking, the abnormal tissue can be removed (excisional techniques) or it can be destroyed (ablative techniques). Removing the entire transformation zone

Table 3.1 Comparison of excisional and ablative techniques for removing abnormal tissue

Technique	Description
Excisional	
LLETZ	Removal of the transformation zone using an electrodiathermy loop (or needle). Can usually be done under local anaesthesia
Laser cone	Removal of the transformation zone using the laser as a 'knife'. Can usually be done under local anaesthesia
Knife cone biopsy	Performed under general anaesthesia
Hysterectomy	The ultimate excision. May be suitable if the woman has other gynaecological problems
Ablative	
Radical electrodiathermy	Burning the transformation zone. Usually performed under general anaesthesia
Cold-coagulation	A misnomer really, since the tissue is boiled by applying a probe heated to 100–120°C. Performed under local anaesthetic
Cryocautery	Freezes the tissue. Can be performed without anaesthetic
Laser	Vaporises tissue. Can usually be performed under local anaesthesia

has the advantage of allowing a large specimen to be examined: the pathologist can comment on the most severe abnormality and can assess whether all the abnormal tissue has been removed. Destroying the transformation zone does not allow this, so it is mandatory to establish the diagnosis by taking a small biopsy before treatment. However, punch biopsy has been shown to be an inaccurate investigation when compared with subsequent loop excision from the same cervix (Table 3.1).[18]

In terms of how effective the different treatment modalities are, they all achieve a 90–95% cure rate (defined by a normal smear six months after treatment) except cryocautery, which has a cure rate of about 85%.[19]

Glandular premalignancy of the cervix: adenocarcinoma *in situ*

Glandular premalignancy of the cervix is far less common than squamous premalignancy (about 100 times less so) and is neither reliably screened for with cytology nor does it have any particular colposcopic features. The aetiological factors are the same as for squamous lesions and the two coexist in about two-thirds of cases (Figure 3.7). Compared with squamous lesions, HPV-18 is found in a higher proportion of cases. Most pathologists agree that glandular precancer can be divided into low-grade

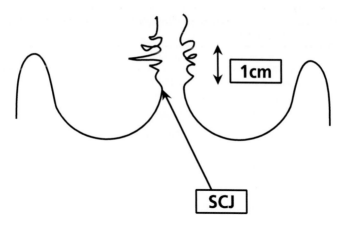

Figure 3.7 Glandular intraepithelial neoplasia; SJC = squamocolumnar junction

TERMINOLOGY	
CIN	Cervical intraepithelial neoplasia: graded 1–3 depending on severity
VAIN	Vaginal intraepithelial neoplasia: graded 1–3 depending on severity
VIN	Vulval intraepithelial neoplasia: graded 1–3 depending on severity
AIS	Adenocarcinoma *in situ*, preinvasive disease of glandular tissue
CIGN	Cervical intraepithelial glandular neoplasia: preinvasive disease of glandular tissue graded low and high grade

and high-grade but there is more debate about whether one can distinguish three groups as in CIN (see Chapter 2). High-grade CIGN is adenocarcinoma *in situ* (AIS). Most of these lesions arise within 1 cm of the squamocolumnar junction but 'skip' lesions are occasionally (< 15%) reported. Despite the latter, the condition can still be amenable to local treatment provided a large enough cone biopsy is taken (> 25 mm) and that the endocervical margins are free from disease. Recurrence of disease occurs in 42% of women with involved endocervical margins and 15% of women with clear margins. Follow-up of women with conservatively treated AIS must include careful endocervical cytological sampling.[20]

VULVAL INTRAEPITHELIAL NEOPLASIA

Premalignant changes are also recognised in other lower genital tract epithelium. Vulval premalignancy or VIN is graded in a similar manner to

Table 3.2 Comparison of features of vulval (*VIN*) and cervical intraepithelial neoplasia (*CIN*)

Similarity	VIN3	CIN3
Proportion of cases of disease adjacent to malignancy	25%	> 90%
Invasive potential	Lower (<10%)	Significant (40%)
Time to progress to invasion	20–30 years	10–15 years
Spontaneous regression	Up to 40%	Low

CIN with grades 1–3 in increasing severity of abnormal cell maturation and stratification (see Chapter 2). However, there are some striking differences between VIN and CIN (Table 3.2).

VIN is not a common disease but it appears to be increasing particularly in younger women (although part of the reason for this may be more effective detection rather than a genuine increase).[21] The association with HPV infection is strong (although not as strong as for CIN) particularly in young women and these women may have other intraepithelial neoplasias of the anogenital tract (a 'field change'). VIN mainly affects the labia minora and the perineum and can take a variety of forms, which accounts for the difficulty in diagnosis. The woman may complain of itching (vulval pruritus), in about 40% cases, or soreness and burning.[22] A substantial number, however, will be asymptomatic and the abnormality will be a chance finding on examination. The lesions may be unifocal or multifocal and there may be extension to the perianal and anal mucosa (Figure 3.8; plate 4).

Diagnosis is made by examining the vulva with a good light source (possible with the colposcope at low magnification). Acetic acid may be used but the changes take longer to occur than for CIN. Clinical suspicions are confirmed by biopsy. Management has become much more conservative in view of the relatively low invasive potential and the physical and psychological scarring that will be inflicted with extensive vulval surgery. Unfortunately, current treatments for VIN are suboptimal in terms of their poor clinical response rates and high relapse rates. The high recurrence rates following many therapies may reflect the fact that they fail to remove the reservoir of HPV present in the vulval skin. Low-grade VIN should be observed. VIN3 lesions can be treated by local excision or laser vaporisation. Recurrences of 39% and 70% have been described after surgical excision and laser ablation, respectively.[23,24] If a woman has VIN, the rest of the lower genital tract should be carefully examined, as there is an increased risk of intraepithelial neoplasia at other sites.

VAGINAL INTRAEPITHELIAL NEOPLASIA

VAIN is extremely uncommon (about 150 times less common than CIN). In 70% of cases of VAIN there will be associated CIN. The average age of the woman with VAIN tends to be greater than for CIN. The major predisposing factor is the same, namely oncogenic HPV, but the reason for the lower incidence is the relative stability of the epithelium compared with the metaplastic cervical epithelium. Women exposed to stilboestrol *in utero* have a higher incidence of VAIN as, here, the areas of metaplastic transformation extend on to the vagina. Around 25% of women with VAIN will have had a hysterectomy previously, either for CIN or benign conditions. Like CIN, VAIN is graded 1–3 but, in common with VIN, the invasive potential is less than for CIN. Treatment of VAIN3 is by surgical excision. This may necessitate a combined abdominovaginal approach to excise the vaginal vault. Chemosurgery using 5-fluorouracil prior to diathermy ablation is an experimental treatment that has shown some promising results. Radiotherapy is an alternative treatment for women who may not be suitable for surgery. Lower grades can be observed. For women who have had hysterectomy where VAIN is seen at the vaginal vault, there may still be disease buried above the vault in the cuff that was closed over at hysterectomy.

SUMMARY
- CIN has a long natural history.
- HPV infection is extremely common but rarely causes cancer.
- Organised cervical cytology screening is effective in reducing the incidence of cervical cancer but is very expensive and may cause significant psychological morbidity.
- Screening is not justified for teenagers.
- Local treatment for CIN is highly effective.
- Vaginal and vulval intraepithelial neoplasias are much less common and appear to have less invasive potential than CIN.

References

1. Koss LG, Stewart FW, Foote FW, *et al*. Some histological aspects of the behaviour of epidermoid carcinoma *in situ* and related lesions of the uterine cervix. *Cancer* 1963; **16**: 1160.

2. McIndoe WA, McLean MR, Jones RW, Mullins PR. The invasive potential of carcinoma *in situ* of the cervix. *Obstet Gynecol* 1984; **64**: 451–8.

3. Richart RM. Natural history of cervical intraepithelial neoplasia. *Clin Obstet Gynecol* 1967; **10**: 748–84.

4. Robertson JH, Woodend BE, Crozier EH, Hutchinson J. Risk of cervical cancer associated with mild dyskaryosis. *BMJ* 1988; **297**: 18–21.

5. Soutter WP. The management of a mildly dyskaryotic smear: immediate referral to colposcopy is safer. *BMJ* 1994; **309**: 591–2.

6. Koutsky L Epidemiology of genital human papillomavirus infection. *Am J Med* 1997; **102**(5A): 3–8.

7. Young LS, Bevan IS, Johnson MA, Blomfield PI, Bromidge T, Maitland NJ, *et al.* The polymerase chain reaction: a new epidemiological tool for investigating cervical human papillomavirus infection. *BMJ* 1989; **298**: 14–18.

8. Syrjanen K, Syrjanen S. Epidemiology of human papilloma virus infections and genital neoplasia. *Scand J Infect Dis* 1990; 69 **Suppl**: 7–17.

9. Alloub MI, Barr BB, McLaren KM, Smith IW, Bunney MH, Smart GE. Human papillomavirus infection and cervical intraepithelial neoplasia in women with renal allografts. *BMJ* 1992; **298**: 153–6.

10. Werness BA, Levine AJ, Howley PM. Association of human papillomavirus types 16 and 18 E6 proteins with p53. *Science* 1990; **248**: 76–9.

11. White E. p53 guardian of Rb. *Nature* 1994; **371**: 21–2.

12. National Health Service Cervical Screening Programme, England: 1997–98 Department of Health Statistical Bulletin 1999 (2), January 1999.

13. Hakama M, Miller AB, Day NE. *Screening for Cancer of the Uterine Cervix.* Lyon: IARC; 1986.

14. Van Wijngaarden WJ, Duncan ID. Rationale for stopping cervical screening in women over 50. *BMJ* 1993; **306**: 967–7.

15. Evaluation of Cervical Cytology. Summary. Evidence Report/Technology Assessment: Number 5, January 1999. Agency for Health Care Policy and Research, Rockville, MD [www.ahrq.gov/clinic/epcsums/cervsumm.htm].

16. National Health Service Cervical Screening Programme, England: 2000–01 Department of Health Statistical Bulletin 2001 (22), September 2001.

17. Marteau TM, Walker PB, Giles J, Smail M. Anxieties in women undergoing colposcopy. *Br J Obstet Gynaecol* 1990; **97**: 859–61.

18. Buxton EJ, Luesley DM, Shafi MI, Rollason T. Colposcopically directed punch biopsy: a potentially misleading investigation. *Br J Obstet Gynaecol* 1991; **98**: 1273–6.

19. Martin-Hirsch PL, Paraskevaidis E, Kitchener H. Surgery for cervical intraepithelial neoplasia. *Cochrane Database Syst Rev* 2001; (4).

20. Etherington IJ, Luesley DM. Adenocarcinoma *in situ* of the cervix: controversies in diagnosis and treatment. *Journal of Lower Genital Tract Diseases* 2001; **5**: 94–8.

21. Jones RW, Baranyai J, Stables S. Trends in squamous cell carcinoma of the vulva: the influence of vulvar intraepithelial neoplasia. *Obstet Gynecol* 1997; **90**: 448–52.

22. Campion MJ, Singer A. Vulvar intraepithelial neoplasia: clinical review. *Genitourinary Med* 1987; **63**: 147–52.

23. DiSaia PJ, Rich WM. Surgical approach to multifocal carcinoma *in situ* of the vulva. *Am J Obstet Gynecol* 1981; **140**: 136–45.

24. Townsend DE, Levine RU, Richart RM, Crum CP, Petrilli ES. Management of

vulvar intraepithelial neoplasia by carbon dioxide laser. *Obstet Gynecol* 1982; **60**: 49–52.

4 Presentation, investigation and diagnosis

Introduction

The division between diagnostic or investigative procedures and treatment is somewhat arbitrary in gynaecological oncology. For some patients, the diagnostic procedure performed may itself be curative; for example stage Ia1 carcinoma of the cervix and stage 1a carcinoma of the vulva. In most cases, the investigations are used not only to make the diagnosis but also to formulate a treatment plan for the individual patient. In the course of investigation and diagnosis, the FIGO stage of the tumour will be documented (see Appendix 1).

Some of the investigations that are routinely used to aid treatment planning, such as magnetic resonance imaging (MRI) in cervical cancer, cannot be used to assign a tumour to a FIGO stage. Although assigning the FIGO stage is important, planning the appropriate management for each individual patient takes priority. This chapter sets out the FIGO staging for each cancer and discusses some of the additional investigations that are used routinely in practice.

Cervical cancer

PRESENTATION

Although the cervical screening programme was not implemented to detect cervical cancer, asymptomatic cases may be detected as a result of screening. Cervical cancer can also arise during the interval between smears in women participating in the cervical screening programme.

Women with postcoital, intermenstrual or persistent vaginal bleeding, or whose cervix looks (Figure 4.1; plate 4) or feels abnormal, should be referred for assessment, even if they are participating in the National Screening Programme. It is worth stressing that adenocarcinomas (i.e. arising from the glandular epithelium) are not only difficult to detect using the current screening programme but also appear to be demonstrating a true increase in incidence.

INVESTIGATION

The majority of patients with suspected cervical cancer are referred to colposcopy clinics.

The detailed description of colposcopic appearances associated with malignancy is beyond the scope of this chapter, but the presence of abnormal blood vessel patterns, an irregular surface contour or the presence of a large lesion would raise the index of suspicion. If invasive

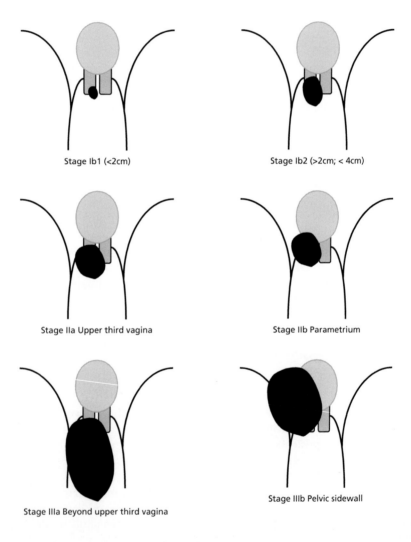

Stage Ib1 (<2cm)

Stage Ib2 (>2cm; < 4cm)

Stage IIa Upper third vagina

Stage IIb Parametrium

Stage IIIa Beyond upper third vagina

Stage IIIb Pelvic sidewall

Figure 4.2 Cervical staging schematic

disease is suspected, then a biopsy of the lesion is obtained. The biopsy may include the whole lesion if small (or subclinical), or simply be representative of a larger, clinically obvious tumour. If there is a large, clinically obvious tumour, an attempt at excising the whole lesion by knife or loop cone should be avoided. These biopsy types do not enhance diagnostic accuracy but may cause haemorrhage or a prolonged inflammatory reaction, leading to difficulties in imaging assessment and delays in definitive treatment.

Following histological confirmation, investigations focus on staging and treatment planning.

The staging of cervical cancer is clinical and must not be changed because of subsequent findings. The following examinations are permitted by FIGO to assign a clinical stage to carcinoma of the cervix (Figure 4.2):

- palpation, inspection and colposcopy of the cervix
- endocervical curettage, hysteroscopy, cystoscopy and proctoscopy
- intravenous urography (see Figure 12.1 on page 121)
- X-ray examination of the lungs and skeleton.

Treatment planning in most centres in the UK often involves other imaging modalities such as computed tomography (CT) or MRI scanning, but these are not considered in allocating a FIGO stage. Where available, MRI scanning has been shown to be superior to clinical staging in assessing the extent of the disease.[1]

In patients who undergo surgery, histopathological examination is used to assess the requirement for adjuvant therapy.

Endometrial cancer

SIGNS AND SYMPTOMS

Postmenopausal bleeding is the most common complaint in patients in whom endometrial cancer is diagnosed (Figure 4.3; plate 5). Around 90% of patients are diagnosed over the age of 50 years, and postmenopausal bleeding is associated with an underlying carcinoma in up to 10% of patients. While commonly associated with older women, endometrial cancer can occur in younger women and may present with irregular or intermenstrual bleeding.

With reference to the cervical screening programme, occasionally cells are detected that may suggest the presence of endometrial pathology.

Because of the strong aetiological association with oestrogenic stimulation, the diagnosis should be considered in symptomatic younger patients with polycystic ovary syndrome, those with irregular bleeding on hormone replacement therapy or those taking tamoxifen. As discussed in Chapter 1, tamoxifen stimulates ovarian oestrogen biosynthesis and elevates plasma oestrogen levels, increasing the risk of endometrial cancer.

INVESTIGATION

The initial investigations are often performed on an outpatient basis and, in many units, dedicated rapid access clinics have been established to investigate postmenopausal bleeding.

Transvaginal scan (TVS) to assess the endometrial thickness is commonly used as a screening tool. If the overall thickness of the endometrium is 5 mm or less and the ovaries appear normal on the scan, then the probability of endometrial cancer is low. The pre-test risk of endometrial cancer for those with postmenopausal bleeding is reduced from 10% to 1% in those with a normal transvaginal scan.[2]

Endometrial biopsies can be obtained as an outpatient using a variety of different sampling devices (Figure 4.4; plate 5). Some units use outpatient hysteroscopy as the screening investigation, combined with endometrial biopsy if indicated. In cases where pathology is suspected, or if the outpatient biopsy is unsatisfactory, then inpatient hysteroscopy combined with dilatation and curettage is performed.

Once the histological diagnosis is confirmed, further investigations include a chest X-ray, assessment of the renal tract (ultrasound or intravenous urography), full blood count and biochemical profile.

Although ultrasound scanning allows some indication of the depth of myometrial invasion, MRI is the optimal imaging modality for this purpose.[3] In addition, the status of the pelvic and para-aortic lymph nodes can be assessed using MRI.

This information is used for treatment planning. The current practice in the UK is for patients to undergo a laparotomy unless they are unfit for surgery or in clinical stage III or IV.

The laparotomy includes peritoneal washings, total abdominal hysterectomy, bilateral salpingo-oophorectomy and pelvic/para-aortic lymph node sampling.

The ASTEC study is currently evaluating the role of pelvic lymphadenectomy in endometrial cancer and is discussed further in Chapter 7.

Ovarian cancer

SIGNS AND SYMPTOMS

Seventy-five percent of patients with ovarian cancer present with advanced disease (stage III or IV). The description of ovarian cancer as a 'silent' disease is a testimony to the insidious nature of the disease; around 15% of patients remain asymptomatic at diagnosis. The symptoms are often vague and most reflect the effect of the tumour filling the pelvis/abdomen:

- abdominal distension
- pressure effects upon bladder/rectum
- dyspnoea
- gastrointestinal symptoms (often of indigestion or mimicking irritable bowel syndrome).

Abnormal vaginal bleeding (sometimes postmenopausal bleeding) is common and may be caused by increased oestrogen production by some tumours due to the increase in ovarian stroma.

In patients with stage I ovarian cancer, the only physical sign is that of a mass arising from the pelvis, unless ascites is present in patients with stage Ic disease.

It is not uncommon, at first presentation, to find a patient with a distended abdomen caused by tumour or ascites (Figure 4.5; plate 6). Cachexia, at initial presentation, is uncommon and patients with advanced disease often look surprisingly well. An omental 'cake' may be palpable in the upper abdomen and a combined vaginal and rectal examination can reveal tumour infiltration of the pouch of Douglas.

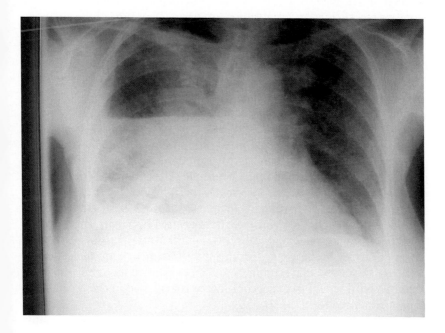

Figure 4.6 Large pleural infusion

There may be enlarged inguinal or cervical lymph nodes. Hepatomegaly is uncommon. For some patients, the first clue to the diagnosis may come with the discovery of a deep vein thrombosis.

Breathlessness may indicate a pleural effusion (Figure 4.6). Because of the vague nature of the symptoms and signs of ovarian cancer, clinicians must be vigilant to the possible presence of an ovarian tumour.

DISSEMINATION OF THE DISEASE

Epithelial ovarian cancer spreads:

- directly to the uterus and fallopian tubes
- via the peritoneum to the rest of the peritoneal cavity, especially the omentum
- via the lymphatics to pelvic and para-aortic lymph nodes
- by haematogenous spread to the liver and other organs.

INVESTIGATIONS

Routine investigations for patients with suspected epithelial ovarian cancer should include an ultrasound examination of the abdomen and pelvis, a full blood count, biochemical profile and serum CA125 estimation, as well as a chest X-ray. Other imaging modalities may be appropriate, such as an intravenous urogram, CT or MRI of the abdomen and pelvis. Breast, bronchus, stomach and large bowel cancers often spread to the ovaries. Barium studies or endoscopy should be performed in those suspected of having a primary gastrointestinal malignancy.

Although not part of the FIGO staging, preoperative assessment with CT or MRI can be valuable. Preoperative CT scanning is being used to develop models for predicting resectability of advanced ovarian tumours.[4]

Although raised in the majority of patients with ovarian cancer, the level of serum CA125 *per se* is of no prognostic significance when measured at the time of diagnosis. Measured serially, it aids assessment of response to chemotherapy and, if normalised with treatment, a rise is highly suggestive of recurrent disease.[5]

The FIGO staging for primary ovarian carcinoma is surgical but also includes histological and cytological findings (see Appendix 1).

Accurate staging of ovarian cancer is important – for patients with stage Ia or Ib disease surgery may be the only treatment required. There is evidence to suggest that staging should be performed by those who have expertise in the field of gynaecological oncology, within the setting of a multidisciplinary team.

For further information, see Chapter 10, Ovarian Cancer Standards of Care.

Vulval cancer

SIGNS AND SYMPTOMS

The most common symptom associated with vulval cancer is pruritus. Less commonly, bleeding or the complaint of a lump or ulcer leads to the diagnosis being made. Such symptoms, particularly in older women, make careful examination of the lower genital tract mandatory. A raised 'warty' or ulcerated lesion may be apparent, possibly arising in a background of abnormal vulval skin (Figure 4.7; plate 6) (suggestive of conditions such as vulval intraepithelial neoplasia or lichen sclerosus). Because of the risk of multicentric disease throughout the lower genital tract (discussed in Chapter 3), careful examination of the vagina and cervix must be performed, including cervical cytology (see Chapter 13).

SUMMARY

Cervical cancer
- Patients with postcoital, intermenstrual or persistent vaginal bleeding, or a clinically abnormal cervix should be referred for assessment.
- Staging of cervical cancer is clinical.

Endometrial cancer
Postmenopausal bleeding must always be investigated.
Endometrial cancer does occur in younger women – link with oestrogenic stimulation, e.g. polycystic ovary syndrome, obesity, tamoxifen.

Ovarian cancer
Vigilance required as symptoms may be vague.
75% have advanced disease at diagnosis.
Exclude other primary tumours, such as bowel.

Vulval cancer
Examine patients with vulval symptoms.
Refer early for specialist opinion and biopsy.
Vaginal and cervical assessment required (multicentric disease).

INVESTIGATIONS

For patients with suspect vulval lesions, a biopsy is required to confirm the histological diagnosis. For lesions less than 2 cm in diameter, the biopsy should include a 1 cm margin of normal tissue around the lesion. For larger lesions, diagnostic biopsies should be obtained, including the junction of the lesion and surrounding epithelium (see Chapter 13). In addition, a full blood count, biochemical profile and chest X-ray are recommended baseline investigations.

Following the histological confirmation of squamous carcinoma of the vulva, the further management plan should be determined in a gynaecological cancer centre. The treatment of patients with vulval cancer is individualised on the basis of factors such as the extent of the disease and the patient's general health. Such management plans are often formulated at multidisciplinary meetings, as in some cases preoperative radiotherapy may be indicated (for example to try and reduce the size of a primary lesion to allow preservation of the anal sphincter).

References

1. Hawnaur JM, Johnson RJ, Carrington BM, Hunter RD. Predictive value of clinical examination, transrectal ultrasound and magnetic resonance imaging prior to radiotherapy in carcinoma of the cervix. *Br J Radiol* 1998; **71**: 819–27.

2. Smith-Bindman R, Kerlikowski K, Feldstein VA, Subak L, Scheidler J, Segal M, *et al*. Endovaginal ultrasound to exclude endometrial cancer and other endometrial abnormalities. *JAMA* 1998; **280**: 1510–17.

3. Hardesty LA, Sumkin JH, Hakim C, Johns C, Nath M. The ability of helical CT to preoperatively stage endometrial carcinoma. *Am J Roentgenol* 2001; **176**: 603–6.

4. Bristow RE, Duska LR, Lambrou NC, Fishman EK, O'Neill MJ, Trimble J, *et al*. A model for predicting surgical outcome in patients with advanced ovarian carcinoma using computed tomography. *Cancer* 2000; **89**: 1532–40.

5. Tuxen MK, Soletormos G, Dombernowsky P. Serum tumour marker CA125 in monitoring of ovarian cancer during first line therapy. *Br J Cancer* 2001; **84**: 1301–7.

5 Surgical principles

Introduction

Surgery has various applications in the management of cancer. These roles may change according to the site and extent of the tumour, the general health of the individual and the patient's wishes. In general, the roles that can be performed by surgery include:

- diagnosis
- staging
- treatment
- reconstruction
- palliation.

Diagnosis

In general, the diagnosis of a cancer will be made by means of a biopsy taken either as an outpatient procedure or under general anaesthesia, such as hysteroscopy, cervical biopsy or vulval biopsy. This investigation may also incorporate part of the staging procedure. However, for ovarian cancer the definitive diagnosis may be confirmed only at laparotomy or when the histology results from laparotomy are available. Sometimes the diagnosis is made by means of interventional radiology, e.g. core biopsy of a distant metastasis.

Staging

Staging is a process whereby the extent of the disease at presentation is defined using agreed international guidelines. Most gynaecologists use the FIGO staging system (see Appendix 1), but the TNM system (tumour, nodes, metastases) is also used, particularly with vulval cancer (see Chapter 13). Staging may be clinical or surgical. Clinical staging includes:

- examination under anaesthetic
- tumour biopsy
- cystoscopy (± biopsy)
- sigmoidoscopy (± biopsy)

- endometrial curettage
- chest X-ray
- intravenous urogram
- skeletal X-ray.

Cervical cancer is clinically staged (see Chapter 4) because a significant number of patients will not undergo surgery. Endometrial, ovarian and vulval cancer are surgically staged and therefore the surgical findings, such as nodal status, may be included in the stage.

Although CT and MRI scans may be of value in preoperative assessment, they are not included in the staging procedures. If they were included, hospitals and countries without these facilities would not be able to stage and have meaningful figures for comparison with other countries. Hence, staging is a language for allowing such comparisons and evaluating differing treatment modalities. It also helps in planning treatment and gives some indication of prognosis. In cervical cancer surgical findings, for instance, involved lymph nodes do not alter the staging but may affect management.

Treatment

Surgery is the primary treatment modality in the majority of early stage gynaecological cancers and may have an adjunctive role in more advanced cancer such as ovarian cancer.

Reconstruction

This may be as part of primary surgery, for example at the time of vulvectomy or may be delayed, such as after bowel resection for ovarian carcinoma.

Palliation

While there are many methods of palliation available that avoid the morbidity of surgery, there are circumstances in which the most effective long-term palliation is surgery, for instance in patients with intestinal obstruction caused by ovarian cancer. Although surgical treatment of cancer is aimed at cure and may be considered to have failed in its intent if cure is not achieved, it may provide significant palliation even in these circumstances. Palliation is considered in Chapter 15.

Complications of laparotomy

All abdominal procedures carry risk. The risks associated with surgery for cancer may be due to the procedures necessary to remove the tumour or

Table 5.1   Intraoperative complications of laparotomy

Complication	Cause
Haemorrhage	Especially from the infundibulopelvic ligaments or the bed of an incompletely resected pelvic tumour, which may require direct pressure, the use of a haemostatic substance e.g. Surgicel® (Ethicon), or even internal iliac artery ligation
Bowel damage	Due to direct tumour involvement or adhesion formation
Ureteric or bladder damage	Due to close proximity to tumour or tumour spread
Damage to large blood vessels	Compression or infiltration of external iliac arteries and veins
Direct trauma to other intraabdominal organs	On resection of metastases or due to retraction

a direct result of the cancer itself. Intraoperative problems are detailed in Table 5.1 and postoperative complications in Table 5.2.

Ovarian carcinoma

See also Chapter 10, Ovarian cancer standards of care.

PRIMARY SURGERY

The aim of primary surgery for ovarian cancer is to confirm the diagnosis, stage the disease and remove all of the cancer or optimally cytoreduce or debulk the cancer (i.e., the amount of cancer is removed to an optimum level, which can vary).

At primary surgery, total abdominal hysterectomy, bilateral salpingo-

Table 5.2   Postoperative complications

Complication	Treatment
Ileus	Intraoperative nasogastric tube insertion is advised
Wound dehiscence or incisional hernia	Mass closure is advised
Wound infection	Give prophylactic antibiotics
Deep vein thrombosis and pulmonary embolism	Decrease risk by adequate hydration, thromboembolism-deterrent stockings, thromboprophylaxis and early mobilisation

oophorectomy, omentectomy, retroperitoneal lymph node sampling and peritoneal biopsies should be undertaken and peritoneal washings or ascitic fluid should be obtained for cytology. The surgery should usually be performed through an extended midline incision. Poor outcome in early-stage ovarian cancer is often due to understaging of the disease at initial laparotomy.[1] Care must be taken to avoid intraoperative spillage that may convert stage Ia disease to stage Ic, although the prognostic significance of this is uncertain. In young women in whom the diagnosis is uncertain and who wish to retain their fertility, more conservative surgery is an option. Germ cell tumours are relatively more common in women under 30 years of age and these can be treated with conservative surgery, enabling fertility to be retained.[2] However, young women who opt for conservative surgery at the outset must be aware that the finding of an epithelial ovarian cancer is likely to result in them requiring a further laparotomy.

For stage I disease, surgery alone results in an excellent prognosis, with a greater than 90% five-year survival.

In more advanced ovarian cancer, laparotomy and debulking of the tumour have been considered to be the mainstay of treatment since the work of Griffiths, who reported increased survival in women with residual disease of less than 1.6 cm in diameter compared with those who had bulky residual disease.[3] This has resulted in an increasing acceptance of radical surgery. There have been no randomised controlled trials comparing debulking surgery with no debulking surgery. A meta-analysis of observational studies showed that cytoreductive surgery had only a minimal effect on survival and that the major influence was the type of chemotherapy employed.[4] It has been suggested that the apparent difference in survival in patients who were optimally debulked may be a result of inherent biological characteristics, allowing complete surgical cytoreduction and at the same time enabling longer survival.[5]

Radical surgery is not without its morbidity and risks.[6] In addition, Potter et al. reported on patients in whom bowel resection was undertaken in order to achieve optimal cytoreduction and noted poorer survival than in patients left with residual disease and not undergoing bowel resection.[7] It is therefore appropriate that surgical cytoreduction should be performed in a gynaecological cancer centre without bowel resection unless obstruction is present or imminent. In some circumstances, primary surgery will be for relief of symptoms and diagnosis but have a minimal curative role, for instance when bowel obstruction is present and the patient is too sick for major cytoreductive surgery.

INTERVAL SURGERY

It has been suggested that if optimal debulking surgery is not achieved at primary surgery, a further attempt at surgery halfway through chemotherapy may improve survival. Patients with progressive disease are excluded from further surgery. A study by van der Burg demonstrated a six-months median improvement in survival of patients undergoing interval surgery.[8] The cost benefit of this interval procedure is not yet clear and further studies are in progress to attempt to confirm the benefits of interval surgery.

There is also currently interest in the role of timing of surgery. The diagnosis of advanced ovarian cancer can be made reliably by either CT scan and scan-guided fine needle biopsies[9] or by open laparoscopy.[10] A number of studies have proposed chemotherapy prior to definitive surgery in patients with advanced ovarian carcinoma. Surwit et al.[11] reported on 29 patients and Schwartz et al.[12] described the management of 59 patients and proposed that survival was no different from a group of patients treated by primary cytoreductive surgery. Randomised prospective trials are required to establish the role of delayed primary surgery in patients with stage III ovarian carcinoma. However, it does already have a role in patients who are unfit for surgery or with stage IV disease.

SECOND-LOOK SURGERY

This has now been largely abandoned in UK practice. The aim of this surgery was to establish when chemotherapy could be stopped or alternative treatment introduced. A large prospective randomised study in 1988 showed that routine second-look laparotomy did not alter survival rates and should be abandoned.[13]

SURGERY AT RELAPSE

In this context there is some evidence that young women who have undergone optimum primary therapy and a treatment-free interval of 12 months were more likely to have optimal second surgery with an improved median survival.[14] A significant number of women with recurrent disease will develop bowel obstruction and surgery is often the palliation method of choice.

Cervical cancer

This cancer is staged clinically by means of an examination under anaesthetic, cystoscopy, sigmoidoscopy, chest X-ray and imaging of the renal tract. Increasing numbers of women are presenting with very early (stage Ia) disease diagnosed at the time of a loop biopsy of the cervix and these patients may not require formal staging, provided that the disease has been completely excised. After a patient has been staged, this information is used to decide the most appropriate treatment for that

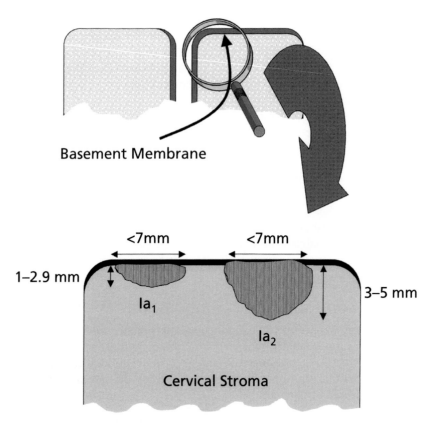

Basement Membrane

<7mm <7mm

1–2.9 mm

Ia_1

Ia_2

3–5 mm

Cervical Stroma

Figure 5.1 Cervical pathalogical substaging

individual patient.

The classification of early stage disease requires careful assessment by the pathologist and is extremely important in treatment planning (Figure 5.1). Patients with stage Ia1 can be treated by loop or cone biopsy of the cervix, thus retaining the potential for fertility. Stage Ia2 can be treated by a large cone biopsy or simple hysterectomy. In this substage, however, there is an increased incidence of lymph node positivity and some would argue that if there is evidence of lymphovascular space involvement, the lymph nodes should also be removed.

Stage Ib disease can be treated by surgery or radiotherapy and the surgical options are:

- radical hysterectomy with bilateral pelvic lymphadenectomy
- radical vaginal hysterectomy and laparoscopic or extraperitoneal lymph node dissection

- radical trachelectomy with laparoscopic or extraperitoneal lymph node dissection.

While these procedures are all considered therapeutic, lymph node dissection may also provide important prognostic information that is not included in staging but may demonstrate that adjuvant radiotherapy is indicated. The removal of enlarged involved lymph nodes may also have a therapeutic role, although this is not fully defined. The surgical options do allow ovarian conservation in young women. The ovaries do not need to be removed routinely in young women and the incidence of metastases in the ovary is low. However, this must be discussed with each patient individually.

Radical hysterectomy differs from a normal hysterectomy in the following ways:

- the uterine vessels are ligated close to their source
- exposure of the ureters to their insertion into the bladder

Table 5.3	Complications of surgical treatment of cervical cancer	
Stage	Surgical treatment	Complications
Ia1	LLETZ	Secondary haemorrhage, due to infection, is treated with bed rest, antibiotics and, occasionally, cervical suturing
	Knife cone biopsy Simple hysterectomy	Complications as for laparotomy
Ia2	Knife cone biopsy Wertheim's hysterectomy and lymph node dissection	See Table 5.4 for complications
	Radical trachelectomy	Vaginal procedure with excision of cervix, upper vagina and parametrium (uterine body is left in situ). Immediate complications are infection and bleeding
Stage Ib1	Wertheim's hysterectomy and lymph node dissection	See Table 5.4 for complications
Stage Ib2	Preoperative chemoradiation and adjuvant hysterectomy	
Stage IIa	Schauta radical vaginal hysterectomy and lymph node dissection	Involves taking a vaginal cuff, often with enlargement of the vaginal orifice with Schuchardt's incision (like a large mediolateral episiotomy). Decreased operative mortality, c.f. Wertheim's, complications as that for vaginal hysterectomy with increased risk of ureteric damage

- excision of the paracervical tissues
- removal of the pelvic side wall lymph nodes
- excision of a vaginal cuff.

The possibility of radical cervical surgery with conservation of the uterine body has been pioneered in France by Dargent[15] and in the UK by Shepherd et al.[16] While there have been successful pregnancies following this form of treatment, long-term follow-up is not yet available, although early results are encouraging.

In relapsed cervical cancer, radical exenterative surgery has a role for small central recurrences. However, this surgery has a high morbidity and should only be considered after multidisciplinary discussion. Only a team with the appropriate experience of this major surgery and the postoperative management of these patients should perform it. The mortality varies from 6–24% and the five-year survival varies from 20–50%. There has also been a move towards reanastomosis of the bowel to avoid permanent colostomy and the development of continent urinary conduits.

COMPLICATIONS OF SURGICAL TREATMENT

There are some complications associated with surgical treatment of cervical cancer. These are listed in Table 5.3. Radical hysterectomy is considered a more morbid procedure than a simple hysterectomy. The complications that may occur during or following radical hysterectomy are shown in Table 5.4.

Endometrial cancer

The standard surgical management for endometrial cancer in the UK has been total abdominal hysterectomy and bilateral salpingo-oophorectomy. However, complete FIGO staging requires a full laparotomy, peritoneal washings for cytology and pelvic or para-aortic lymph node sampling. If the cervix is involved, a radical hysterectomy is required to ensure adequate excision of tumour.

While the majority of patients with endometrial carcinoma have an excellent prognosis after hysterectomy and bilateral salpingo-oophorectomy, the overall five-year survival is only 65%. Lymphadenectomy is indicated in cases of endometrial carcinoma in which the nodes are macroscopically enlarged but there have been no randomised surgical trials of routine pelvic lymphadenectomy in this disease. When fully staged surgically, 22% of patients with clinical stage I disease have extrauterine disease in the form of positive peritoneal washings, nodal disease and/or peritoneal or adnexal spread.[17] While the

Table 5.4 Complications of surgical treatment of cervical cancer

Complication	Cause	Comment
Haemorrhage, particularly at ureteric tunnel, paracolpos and vaginal edge, external iliac artery and vein, obturator fossa, bifurcation of common iliac artery and vein, para-aortic lymph nodes		The use of regional anaesthesia reduces small-vessel oozing
Ureteric dysfunction	Damage to the ureteric blood supply Damage to the ureteric nerve supply Oedema of the wall of the ureter Periureteric infection in the retroperitoneal space	
Ureteric stricture		Develops as a late complication and may require surgery
Ureterovaginal fistulae		Develops as a late complication and may require surgery
Bladder dysfunction	Damage to sympathetic nerves in uterosacral and cardinal ligaments results in bladder hypertonicity due to parasympathetics Oedema of bladder neck and muscle Hypotonicity as a result of overdistension of a hypertonic bladder	Catheterisation for six to eight days postoperatively is recommended
Urinary tract infection		
Vesicovaginal fistulae		
Pelvic lymphocyst at the pelvic brim or pelvic sidewall		May cause pain, obstruction or become infected. May require surgical drainage
Peripheral leg lymphoedema		May develop late and require specialised massage
Nerve damage to the obturator, genitofemoral, femoral, perineal or sciatic nerves		
Sexual dysfunction		Increased if the patient receives adjuvant radiotherapy

overall five-year survival for patients with stage I disease is 90% and for patients with surgical stage I disease is 98%, it falls to 60% in patients with extrauterine disease.[18] However, there is a study in progress in the UK that is seeking to determine both the therapeutic and the prognostic role of lymphadenectomy. There is also controversy over whether this should be a complete node dissection or sampling.

Laparoscopically assisted surgery for endometrial cancer is gaining in popularity and may decrease the morbidity and length of hospital stay for these women. The principal danger of laparoscopic surgery is the risk of injury to bowel, bladder or ureters, but there have been a number of studies suggesting that this is a safe alternative.[19,20] The eventual role of laparoscopic lymphadenectomy in endometrial cancer is likely to be determined by the role defined for lymphadenectomy.

In some patients who are extremely unfit the appropriate management may be vaginal hysterectomy.

Vulval cancer

Biopsy of a vulval lesion is essential for diagnosis prior to definitive surgery. This may be possible as a minor procedure under local anaesthesia or it may be performed under general anaesthesia. When performed under general anaesthesia, the operability of a lesion may be assessed with particular reference to its proximity to the urethra or anus. Alternatively, smaller lesions may be completely excised as an excisional biopsy.

Definitive surgery for vulval cancer consists of radical local excision of the vulval lesion and bilateral inguinal lymphadenectomies. Radical surgery for vulval cancer has excellent cure rates but results in high morbidity with wound breakdown in up to 85% of patients and lymphoedema in 50% of patients.

The morbidity of surgery for vulval cancer has been reduced by the introduction of the triple incision approach to replace the classical *en bloc* butterfly incision (Figure 5.2). This has reduced morbidity (Figures 5.3 and 5.4; plate 7: Figure 5.5; plate 8) with no apparent effect on survival.[21]

The role of inguinal lymphadenectomy in vulval cancer is both diagnostic and therapeutic if the lymph nodes are involved. However, the lymph nodes are involved in only 10% of patients with vulval cancer and in 90% of cases lymphadenectomy is principally for staging and prognosis. Pelvic lymphadenectomy is no longer practised for vulval cancer. Lesions less than 1 mm depth invasion do not require inguinal lymphadenectomy and lateral lesions less than 2 cm in size can be treated by unilateral inguinal lymphadenectomy.[22] There are currently no reliable methods of assessing lymph node status preoperatively, although ultrasound-guided biopsies and sentinel node biopsies are being assessed.

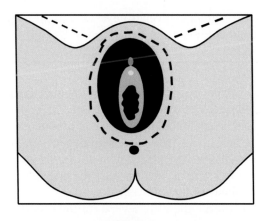

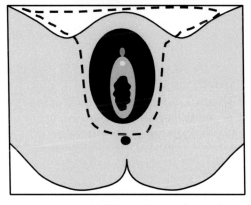

Figure 5.2 Schematic of triple incision vulvectomy and *en bloc* procedure

Surgery for vulval cancer may also involve significant reconstructive surgery, either in the form of local skin flaps (Figure 5.6; plate 8) or with the aid of plastic surgeons' more advanced myocutaneous flaps using rectus abdominis or gracilis muscles. Surgery for vulval cancer may involve resection of part of the urethra or anus and urinary diversion or colostomy may be necessary. In advanced disease, the role of chemoradiotherapy prior to surgery should be considered in order to potentially preserve pelvic anatomy.

SURGERY IN RECURRENT OR ADVANCED DISEASE

Surgery may have a palliative or curative role in advanced or recurrent disease. Patients with localised recurrent disease in the pelvis or abdomen may be suitable for surgical management. This may involve cooperation with colorectal surgeons, urologists or vascular surgeons. Patients should be carefully assessed preoperatively to exclude distant metastases and to establish the potential for curative treatment.

SUMMARY

- Surgery may fulfil many different roles in the management of gynaecological oncology patients.
- Surgery should be tailored to the individual patient.
- In ovarian cancer, surgery may be diagnostic and curative, solely diagnostic or palliative. The ideal timing of surgical intervention and reintervention will vary depending upon the patient's general health and the resectability of their disease.
- In endometrial cancer, there are several controversies as to the extent of surgery required and recruitment to studies is essential to answer these questions.
- Vulval cancer is no longer always treated by radical *en bloc* vulvectomy.
- Conservative surgery should be considered for young patients with early cervical cancer.
- Laparoscopic surgery is playing an increasing role in the management of gynaecological oncology patients.
- Surgery has an important role to play in palliation.

References

1. Venesmaa P. Epithelial ovarian cancer: impact of surgery and chemotherapy on survival during 1977–1990. *Obstet Gynecol* 1994; **84**: 8–11.

2. Abu-Rustum N, Aghajanian C. Management of malignant germ cell tumours of the ovary. *Semin Oncol* 1998; **25**: 235–42.

3. Griffiths CT. Surgical resection of tumour bulk in the primary treatment of ovarian carcinoma. *Natl Cancer Inst Monogr* 1975; **42**: 101–4.

4. Hunter RW, Alexander NDE, Soutter WP. Meta-analysis of surgery in advanced ovarian carcinoma: is cytoreduction an independent determinant of prognosis? *Am J Obstet Gynecol* 1992; **166**: 504–11.

5. Hoskins WJ, McGuire WP, Brady MF, Homesly HD, Creasman WT, Berman M, *et al*. The effects of diameter of largest residual disease on survival after primary cytoreductive surgery in patients with suboptimal residual ovarian carcinoma. *Am J Obstet Gynecol* 1994; **170**: 974–80.

6. Guidozzi F, Ball JHS. Extensive primary cytoreductive surgery for advanced epithelial ovarian cancer. *Gynecol Oncol* 1994; **53**: 326–30.

7. Potter ME, Partridge EE, Hatch KD, Soong SJ, Austin JM, Shingleton HM. Primary surgical therapy of ovarian cancer: how much and when. *Gynecol Oncol* 1991; **40**: 195–200.

8. Van der Burg ME, van Lent M, Buyse M, Kobierska A, Colombo N, Favalli G, *et al*. The effect of debulking surgery after induction chemotherapy on the prognosis in advanced epithelial ovarian cancer. *N Engl J Med* 1995; **332**: 629–34.

9. Nelson BE, Rosenfield AT, Schwartz PE. Pre-operative abdominopelvic computed tomographic prediction of optimal cytoreduction in epithelial ovarian carcinoma. *J Clin Oncol* 1993; **11**: 166–72.

10. Van Dam PA, Decloedt J, Tjama W, Vergote IB. Diagnostic laparoscopy to assess operability of advanced ovarian cancer: a feasibility study. *Eur J Gynaecol Oncol* 1997; **18**: 272–3.

11. Surwit E, Childers J, Atlas M, Nour M, Hatch K, Hallam A, *et al*. Neoadjuvant chemotherapy for advanced ovarian cancer. *Int J Gynecol Cancer* 1996; **6**: 356–61.

12. Schwartz PE, Chambers JT, Makuch R. Neoadjuvant chemotherapy for advanced ovarian cancer. *Gynecol Oncol* 1994; **53**: 33–7.

13. Luesley D, Lawton F, Blackledge G, Hilton C, Kelly R, Rollason T, *et al*. Failure of second-look laparotomy to influence survival in epithelial ovarian cancer. *Lancet* 1988; **ii**: 599–603.

14. Segna RA Dottino PR, Mandeli JP, Konsker K, Cohen CJ, *et al*. Secondary cytoreduction for ovarian cancer following cisplatin therapy. *J Clin Oncol* 1993; **11**: 434–9.

15. Dargent D. Laparoscopic surgery and gynaecologic cancer. *Curr Opin Obstet Gynecol* 1993 ; **5**: 294–300.

16. Shepherd JH, Crawford RAF, Oram DH. Radical trachelectomy: a way to preserve fertility in the treatment of early cervical cancer. *Br J Obstet Gynaecol* 1998; **105**: 912–16.

17. Creasman WT, Morrow CP, Bundy BN, Homeseley HD, Graham JE, Heller PB. Surgical pathologic spread patterns of endometrial cancer. A Gynaecologic Oncology Cancer Group Study. *Cancer* 1987; **60**: 2035–41.

18. Gal D, Recio FO, Zamurovic D. The New International Federation of Obstetrics and Gynaecology surgical staging and survival rates in early endometrial carcinoma. *Cancer* 1992; **69**: 200–2.

19. Holub Z, Voracek J, Shomani A. A comparison of laparoscopic surgery with an open procedure in endometrial cancer. *Eur J Gynaecol Oncol* 1998; **19**: 294–6.

20. Spirtos NM, Schlaerth JB, Gross GM, Spirtos TW, Schlaerth AC, Ballon SC. Cost and quality-of-life analyses of surgery for early endometrial cancer: laparotomy versus laparoscopy. *Am J Obstet Gynecol* 1996; **174**: 1795–9.

21. Hacker NF, Leuchter RS, Berek JS, Castaldo TW, Lagasse LD. Radical vulvectomy and bilateral inguinal lymphadenectomy through separate groin incisions *Obstet Gynecol* 1981; **58**: 574–9.

22. Cavanagh D, Hoffman MS. Controversies in the management of vulvar cancer. *Br J Obstet Gynaecol* 1996; **103**: 293–300.

6 Role of laparoscopic surgery

History of laparoscopic surgery in gynaecological oncology

Jacobaeus first described the use of optical instruments to visualise the peritoneal cavity in 1910. He achieved this by inserting a Nitze cystoscope into a pneumoperitoneum created via a trocar. Following this description the application of laparoscopic surgery in gynaecology stagnated until the late 1930s and the advent of various laparoscopic sterilisation techniques. With the reporting of the use of the laparoscope to manage tubal pregnancies in the early 1980s, interest in how laparoscopic surgical techniques could be applied to gynaecological surgery was rejuvenated and since that time an increasing number of centres have incorporated it into their management of gynaecological malignancies. This was initially championed by the French followed closely by the Americans and is now practised to varying degrees in many countries where gynaecological oncology is regarded as a subspecialty within the framework of general gynaecology.

CERVICAL CANCER

Among the early pioneers in the development of laparoscopic gynaecological oncology was Dargent, who published his group's now famous description of pelvic lymph node dissection in patients with cervical malignancies. This was a modification of the technique that had been developed to dissect out pelvic lymph nodes in prostatic cancer patients; a technique that had been shown to carry a lower morbidity and monetary cost compared with the traditional open technique.

With the realisation that pelvic lymph node dissection could be performed safely and effectively, there was a resurgence of interest in performing radical vaginal hysterectomies for cervical cancer in the early 1990s. This was then extended to a laparoscopic radical abdominal hysterectomy, of varying degrees of radicality, and combined with laparoscopic pelvic node dissection. This level of laparoscopic surgery has only been developed in a small number of centres in France and the USA. It will probably remain so until its true value is proven, as it presents the most skilled endoscopic surgeon with a formidable technical challenge and carries a significant risk of morbidity even in skilled hands. Dargent recognised a potential role for the laparoscope in early cervical cancer patients wishing to preserve fertility. He described the combined approach of laparoscopic lymph node dissection with radical vaginal trachelectomy in the early 1990s. This is a surgical technique that does not present the skilled laparoscopic surgeon with too difficult a challenge and has been shown in case series to offer a reasonable chance of successful pregnancy outcome in appropriately selected patients. An increasing number of cancer centres now offer this type of surgery as part of their oncology service.

ENDOMETRIAL CANCER

The use of laparoscopic surgery for staging of endometrial cancer did not develop as early as it did for cervical cancer because of the initial inability to sample the para-aortic nodes. However, techniques for this level of sampling have been described with a high degree of success in terms of the proportion of patients amenable to this surgery and also lymph node harvest. At present, the value of laparoscopic surgery in the staging of both early and previously unstaged endometrial disease is being evaluated in two GOG studies.

OVARIAN CANCER

The value of laparoscopic surgery in the management of ovarian cancers has been described since the early 1970s, with second-look laparoscopy for patients with advanced ovarian cancer who received chemotherapy and/or surgery very much in vogue. However, the true value of such endoscopic surgery in the management of these patients has never been proven and has virtually ceased in all but a few cases where tissue sampling is required for chemosensitivity testing. In the 1990s, a number of case series concentrated on presumed early-stage ovarian cancer and its management. The results of a Gynaecolgical Oncology Group (GOG) study evaluating the merit of laparoscopic staging in patients with incompletely staged cancers of the ovary (GOG 9302) are awaited. There has also been an increased move towards using an endoscopic approach to the diagnosis of advanced ovarian cancer, particularly with the advent of interval debulking surgery when used in conjunction with chemotherapy. Overall, the value of endoscopic surgery in the management of ovarian cancer patients has not been clarified in an objective way and at present the development of a multicentre study is awaited, to define what is the most appropriate use of this type of surgery in ovarian cancer patients.

Laparoscopic surgery in the management of gynaecological cancers

The management of the three most common gynaecological cancers, ovarian, endometrial and cervical, increasingly includes the use of endoscopic surgery in many Western European countries and the USA. The use of this type of surgery in the management of vulval and vaginal cancers is at a less advanced stage of development and is largely restricted to a few centres in France; for this reason, the latter two cancers are not considered in this chapter.

CERVICAL CANCER

For those patients with stage Ia1 disease, the performance of a cone biopsy either with knife or loop diathermy is all that is required, as long as the margin of the lesion is completely removed and the patient is comfortable with conservative therapy. This reflects the fact that when the depth of invasion is less than 3 mm the risk of metastases is extremely small. When the margins are not confidently clear or the stage is Ia2 then further therapy is necessary. Traditionally, this has either been a repeat cone biopsy, a total abdominal hysterectomy or vaginal hysterectomy, with or without assessment of the pelvic lymph nodes. For the younger patient who wishes to preserve fertility and has a stage Ia2 or even early stage Ib1 cancer, conservative therapy in the form of trachelectomy can be offered. For the older patient, definitive therapy is essential and this involves removal of the cervix and uterus. It can be argued that a vaginal approach is advantageous in this situation, as it allows the lesion extent to be defined. This can be either a routine vaginal hysterectomy or as a laparoscopically assisted vaginal hysterectomy. It is possible that using this route for hysterectomy aids in identifying the 2.5% of patients in whom the transformation zone extends to the fornices of the vagina thereby reducing the risk of residual cytological and histological abnormality.[1]

The major advantage that laparoscopic surgery has in the management of early-stage cervical cancer is in allowing assessment of the pelvic lymph nodes. For those patients with stage Ia1 who wish to have a hysterectomy for coincidental management of other pathologies, such as fibroids or menorrhagia, the standard laparoscopically assisted vaginal hysterectomy will be ideal. The ovaries can be removed or preserved as desired and visual assessment of the lymph nodes can be performed and, where appropriate, sampling can be carried out.

For those patients with stage Ia2, there is a small but significant risk of lymph node metastases. For this reason, laparoscopically assisted vaginal hysterectomy to remove the cervix and uterus and then lymph node sampling or even comprehensive lymphadenectomy can be performed by appropriately trained surgeons without undue difficulty.

PELVIC LYMPHADENECTOMY TECHNIQUE

Pelvic lymphadenectomy is performed laparoscopically by grasping the round ligament, which may be divided if desired, moving the uterus over to the opposite side using an intrauterine manipulator and incising the peritoneum of the pelvic sidewall along the line of the psoas muscle, thereby exposing the external iliac vessel and the infundibulopelvic ligament. The nodes can be removed from the artery, beginning laterally, using the genitofemoral nerve as the lateral limit of the dissection. If the fascia is divided along the line of the artery on the medial side of the genitofemoral nerve, by putting medial tension on the fascia, the entire block of nodes and lymphatic vessels can be completely removed, leaving the artery skeletalised. This procedure is repeated on the iliac vein and then, inferiorly, the obturator nerve and nodes are exposed and these are removed by careful sharp dissection with the aid of diathermy and/or clips. There is no need to close the peritoneum at the end of the procedure and the laparoscopic vaginal hysterectomy can then be performed in the usual way.

It has been recommended that laparoscopic surgery should become the standard therapy in the management of stages Ia1 and Ia2 carcinoma of the cervix. Most surgeons find that node harvest rapidly equals that of the open procedure and the ease of performance and reduction in morbidity by far outweigh any cost disadvantage.[1] However, this is not yet a universally held view in the UK. This is at least partly because there is still a relative lack of the required skill among gynaecologists and also because of the lack of large multicentre, randomised controlled trials that have unequivocally proven a significant advantage for this type of surgery over the more traditional surgical approach. Furthermore, the incidence of lymph node positivity in stage Ia1 disease is small and almost certainly does not justify the additional surgery.

In more advanced cases of cervical cancer, surgery has been used for assessing aortic lymph nodes before undertaking radiotherapy, although this is not routinely performed in the UK. The rate of complications in patients submitted to para-aortic radiotherapy was prohibitive in surgically assessed patients[2] although the use of a retroperitoneal approach significantly reduced the complication rate (3.9% versus 11.5%).[3] Despite the fact that that an extraperitoneal approach reduces complications, iatrogenic morbidity is excessive, considering that the chances of survival are enhanced for only a limited subpopulation and not for the whole population. As a consequence, pretreatment staging surgery disappeared. However, the advent of laparoscopic techniques has completely reversed the situation and in some countries (notably France, Italy and Germany), staging surgery is being used once again in more advanced cases of cervical cancer.[4] In the UK, it is not standard practice to perform para-aortic lymphadenectomy in cervical cancer, as radiotherapy to the para-aortic nodes is not routinely performed in most cancer centres.

For those cases of early cervical cancer who are found to be node-negative, surgery is the appropriate therapy and no further node sampling is required, as the risk of nodal spread to the para-aortic nodes is so small. However, if the patient is found to be node-positive with less than three nodes containing metastases it has been recommended that a systematic lymphadenectomy be performed from the left renal vein down to the femoral ring.[4,5] Interestingly, the same author recommends that, for such surgery, laparotomy is the preferred route because of the marked technical difficulties in performing such a systematic lymphadenectomy laparoscopically.

Apart from laparoscopic lymphadenectomy, the other role that minimal access surgery has to play in the management of cervical cancer is the removal of the central lesion. In the UK, this has traditionally been in the form of a cone biopsy or total abdominal hysterectomy for stage Ia and a Wertheim hysterectomy for more advanced disease where more radical surgery is required. A full laparoscopic radical hysterectomy is an alternative for some surgeons, although once again this has not been performed regularly in the UK and has been more common in Western Europe and the USA. It is a technically difficult procedure to perform, largely because it is difficult to divide the caudal part of the paracervix, due to the large amount of plexoid veins that are present at this level. As a result, the specimens produced at radical laparoscopic hysterectomy are not equivalent to those obtained from other techniques developed from a century of classical radical surgery.[4] An alternative to this technique is to perform a combination of a laparoscopic and a radical vaginal hysterectomy. In this procedure, the laparoscopic part extends to the paracervical resection and the surgery is then completed by performing a proximal type vaginal hysterectomy. This combined laparoscopic–vaginal radical hysterectomy is believed to result in adequate paracervical clearance and a reduced level of bladder associated morbidity and is currently undergoing prospective trials at the cancer centres in Lyon and Roubaix, France.

ENDOMETRIAL CANCER

The use of laparoscopic surgery in the management of endometrial cancer initially concentrated on the surgical staging of the disease and the first reports involved patients with early stage disease in whom the uterus had not yet been removed. These patients underwent surgical staging including a laparoscopically assisted vaginal hysterectomy, salpingo-oophorectomy and lymphadenectomy. The second group of patients were those in whom surgical staging was not performed at the time of their hysterectomy and these patients underwent laparoscopic surgery to obtain peritoneal cytology, remove regional lymph nodes and remove remaining adnexa in some patients. These reports are essentially case series and, to date, there has been no large scale randomised trial comparing laparoscopic and open surgical techniques and their long-term outcomes.

What can be said for laparoscopic surgery in the management of endometrial cancer is that surgical staging can be performed effectively using the laparoscope (including para-aortic lymphadenectomy), a vaginal hysterectomy can be assisted effectively and there is evidence that there is a significant reduction in hospital stay for the patient and, by inference, a reduced recovery time.[6,7] It is also apparent that the learning curve for the laparoscopic lymphadenectomy is fairly short and can be acquired by well trained gynaecological surgeons with an interest in endoscopic surgery.

Defining any extension of the above role that laparoscopic surgery may have will take time and will be heavily dependent upon the survival data being equal to that of open surgery. Such data will take several years to accrue and even then will be hampered by the small numbers involved in the initial studies. It is possible that the results of the ASTEC study that commenced in 1998 in the UK will give some indication of the role that laparoscopic surgery may play in the management of endometrial cancer when these are published.

OVARIAN CANCER

As described above, operative laparoscopy entered the field of gynaecological oncology with the advent of the laparoscopic pelvic lymphadenectomy for the staging of early cervical cancer. Laparoscopic para-aortic lymphadenectomy developed simultaneously in France and the USA and initially was described in a series of case reports for a variety of malignancies including ovarian cancer. Thereafter, a number of case series suggested that this procedure was safe and adequate for the purpose. It was the development of this technique that had a largest impact on the utilisation of endoscopic surgery in the management of ovarian cancer.

Surwit and Childers[8] have described the use of the laparoscope for ovarian cancer management in two settings. The first was in a cohort of patients undergoing second-look laparoscopy. The entire cohort of 40 patients had received chemotherapy following surgical debulking. Interestingly, 10% of these patients were not able to undergo restaging of their disease status due to extensive intraperitoneal adhesions. Significant complications occurred in 14% of these patients, with three patients requiring laparotomy for repair of trauma to the vena cava, repair of a trocar injury to the transverse colon and one to repair a small bowel enterotomy.

The second group consisted of 14 patients with presumed early ovarian cancer, who underwent laparoscopic staging of their disease. Five of these patients had been referred unstaged after their malignant masses had been removed and nine of them had malignant ovarian tumours discovered during the laparoscopic management of their adnexal masses and underwent laparoscopic staging at the time of their primary procedures. Surwit describes no complications within this cohort of patients and all patients were successfully staged according to FIGO criteria.

The same author has described the value of laparoscopic cytoreduction after neoadjuvant chemotherapy for advanced ovarian cancer. In a small series of 11 patients he described how optimal debulking was achieved laparoscopically in patients who had at least a 1-log decrease in their serum CA125 levels and no apparent extensive disease clinically. These patients suffered no major complications as a result of their surgery and had a mean hospital stay of three days and a mean operating time of 1.9 hours. Although this is only a small series it does indicate that laparoscopic surgery may have a role to play in carefully selected patients who are part of an interval debulking surgery treatment protocol.

The role of endoscopic surgery in the management of suspicious adnexal masses has yet to be clarified. To date, there is no universal agreement of the precise role in this clinical setting although guidelines published by the American College of Obstetrics and Gynecology for avoiding unsuspected malignancy in the laparoscopic management of adnexal masses will probably be accepted by most gynaecologists.[9]

The following criteria suggest a low risk of malignancy:

- ultrasound findings of a small mass with thin walls
- no solid parts, no internal echoes, septations or excrescences
- no ascitic fluid in the pelvis
- no family history
- postmenopausal patient should have a normal serum CA125 levels.

Various predictive models for malignancy risk index have been developed using these criteria but the maximum sensitivity that can be achieved is 80–90%. This is still considered too poor a predictor for many centres to allow the use of laparoscopic surgical techniques for all but a small subgroup of patients presenting with adnexal masses. The major reason that there is reluctance to perform laparoscopic surgery in patients with adnexal masses is the fear of rupture and spillage of malignant cysts and their contents; there is a concern that this will worsen the long-term prognosis for that patient. However, few data are available to support the concept that capsular rupture and tumour spill adversely affect prognosis or survival. Only one study[10] has shown a statistically significant difference in five-year survival of patients with stage I ovarian carcinoma who had rupture of the tumour capsule versus unruptured capsules. This was a small retrospective study, the patients were not staged, and tumour grade, tumour adherence and tumour excrescences were not considered in the analysis. Sjovall et al.[11] showed that patients with preoperative rupture had worse survival rates than those with intraoperative rupture (ten-year survival 59% versus 87%), indicating that complete resection of all malignancies at the primary procedure is mandatory. There is no room for tumour spill followed by a delay in definitive management and copious irrigation should be used if spillage occurs. Obviously, spill should be avoided if possible but if a surgeon has the skills to carry out resection and management of ovarian cancer then fear of capsular rupture should not prevent them from managing suspicious adnexal masses laparoscopically.[8] It is not possible, even at laparotomy, to avoid capsular rupture with every suspicious mass, particularly with large and adherent masses, so a varying management protocol is recommended, depending on the surgeon's skills and philosophy on capsular rupture. If a mass can be removed intact then it should be and if it must be drained it can still be managed laparoscopically if the surgeon can drain without spill. If the mass is at risk of rupture because of adherence or because the surgeon considers it unsafe then laparotomy should be used. There is no role for incomplete resection or cyst aspiration in the laparoscopic management of adnexal masses as this could result in delay that increases the risk of recurrence in these patients.

PORT SITE RECURRENCE

Another major concern when laparoscopic surgery is used for gynaecological malignancies is the rate of port site recurrences. Most port site recurrences occur following laparoscopic colectomy for colon cancer or laparoscopic cholecystectomy for gallbladders that contained occult malignancies. In both of these operations cancerous tissue is dragged through a small incision, which, in the majority of cases, receives no further therapy postoperatively. Reported port site recurrences associated with gynaecological cancers have occurred almost exclusively following diagnostic laparoscopy for pelvic masses that subsequently proved to be malignant and were always associated with disseminated disease.[12] It seems from a review of the reported port site recurrences that they result when the malignancy has a propensity to exfoliate cells into the peritoneal cavity and the trocar site remains untreated or the malignancy is refractory to adjuvant therapy. Whether a pneumoperitoneum enhances significantly the inoculation of exfoliated tumour cells is unknown and speculative.

Conclusion

It is important to consider why we may wish to perform gynaecological surgery laparoscopically rather than by more traditional methods that are generally accepted and with which many gynaecologists are familiar. It is essential to realise that most abdominal operations are performed laparoscopically to reduce the pain and discomfort associated with a laparotomy incision, the duration of hospitalisation and the time to full recovery. Laparoscopic surgery is not used to obtain a better primary surgical result, although it is possible that by reducing adhesion formation the laparoscopic approach to gynaecological malignancies may reduce the complications associated with adjunctive therapy such as radiotherapy following radical hysterectomy.

The laparoscopic management of gynaecological cancers is still in its infancy. There are few randomised controlled trials and there is a scarcity of mature data and long-term follow-up series. This is likely to be the case for several years. No doubt new concepts will continue to develop and existing ones will be modified and it is only right to expect this to occur. It is probable that the application of some of endoscopic techniques for cervical, endometrial and ovarian cancer discussed above will become more widely accepted and refined. They are likely to be coupled more closely with advances in imaging techniques and application of developing medical protocols. One must hope that the results of these endeavours will make the treatment of gynaecological cancer much less of an ordeal for patients than it has been in the past.

References

1. Monaghan J. Microinvasive carcinoma of the cervix. In: Querleu D, Childers JM, Dargent D, editors. *Laparoscopic Surgery in Gynaecological Oncology*. Oxford: Blackwell Science; 1999. p. 135–7.

2. Nelson JH Jr, Boyce J, Macasaet M, Lu T, Bohorquez JF, Nicastri AD, *et al*. Incidence, significance and follow-up of para-aortic lymph nodes metastases in late carcinoma of the cervix. *Am J Obstet Gynecol* 1977; **128**: 336–40.

3. Weiser EB, Bundy BN, Hoskins WJ, Heller PB, Whittington RR, DiSaia PJ, *et al*. Extraperitoneal versus transperitoneal selective para-aortic lymphadenectomy in the treatment and surgical staging of advanced cancer (a GOG study). *Gynecol Oncol* 1989; **33**: 283–9.

4. Dargent D. Invasive carcinoma of the cervix. In: Querleu D, Childers JM, Dargent D, editors. *Laparoscopic Surgery in Gynaecological Oncology*. Oxford: Blackwell Science; 1999. p. 138–47.

5. Fuller AF Jr, Elliott N, Kosloff C, Lewis JL Jr. Lymph node metastases from carcinoma of the cervix stages IB and IIA: implications for prognosis and treatment. *Gynecol Oncol* 1982; **13**: 164–74.

6. Childers JM, Surwit EA. Combined laparoscopic and vaginal surgery for the management of two cases of stage 1 endometrial cancer. *Gynecol Oncol* 1993; **45**: 46–51.

7. Melendez T, Harrigal K, Childers JM, Surwit EA. Laparoscopic management of endometrial cancer: the learning experience. *J Laparoscopic Surg* 1997; **1**: 45–9.

8. Surwit EA, Childers JM. Cancer of the ovary. In: Querleu D, Childers JM, Dargent D, editors. *Laparoscopic Surgery in Gynaecological Oncology*. Oxford: Blackwell Science; 1999. p. 155–9.

9. Maiman M, Boyce F, Goldstein SR *et al*. Laparoscopic surgery in the management of ovarian cysts. *Female Patient* 1992; 1716–23.

10. Webb M, Symmonds R. Site of recurrence of cervical cancer after radical hysterectomy. *Am J Obstet Gynecol* 1980; **138**: 813–17.

11. Sjovall K, Nilsson B, Einhorn N. Different types of rupture of the tumour capsule and impact on survival in early ovarian carcinoma. *Int J Gynecol Cancer* 1994; **4**: 333–6.

7 Radiotherapy: principles and applications

Introduction

The therapeutic use of radioactive materials in patients with gynaecological cancer quickly followed the discovery of X-rays by Roentgen in 1895 and radium by the Curies in 1898.

The versatility of today's radiotherapeutic techniques allows treatment to be offered in a variety of settings, ranging from single modality with curative intent to an adjuvant pre- or postoperative setting. Treatment may also be offered for symptom control in a palliative care setting. The multidisciplinary planning of multimodality treatment has become a central part of the management for patients with gynaecological cancer. It is, therefore, important to have an understanding of the basic radiobiological principles underlying radiotherapeutic techniques and of the situations in which they can be applied.

Radiobiology

Radiotherapy uses the damaging effects of ionising radiation upon cellular DNA.

In clinical radiotherapy, X-rays and gamma-rays, together with beta particles, are the commonly used forms of ionising radiation.

Radiotherapy exerts its effects by direct and indirect mechanisms. Direct damage occurs as the result of breaks in the DNA chains or base deletions. Indirect damage is caused by toxic free radicals released by the interaction of radiation with intracellular water.

The following parameters form the basis of radiobiology:

- repair
- reoxygenation
- repopulation
- redistribution.

There are differences in the ability of various cell types to repair the damage caused by radiation. Clinically, this difference can be exploited by fractionating the dose of radiotherapy to increase the lethal damage to tumour cells, while allowing the repair of normal tissues.

During a course of radiotherapy, viable cells will continue to divide. This is the process of repopulation. Thus, in order to eradicate a tumour, a course of radiotherapy must kill not only the original tumour cells but also those formed by repopulation during the treatment period.

Well-oxygenated cells are more susceptible to radiation-induced damage than hypoxic cells. Reoxygenation is the process whereby relatively hypoxic areas of tumours are thought to use the oxygen that is no longer required by the radiosensitive, well-oxygenated cells killed by previous fractions of radiotherapy.

Cells vary in their response to the effects of radiotherapy throughout the cell cycle. Cells in the G1, early S and G2/M phases are highly sensitive, whereas cells in the late S phase are relatively resistant. Fractionation of the dose of radiotherapy exploits this redistribution of cells through the stages of the cell cycle.

Radiotherapy for patients with gynaecological malignancy is usually given either by teletherapy or by brachytherapy. Teletherapy involves the use of radiation whose source is distant from the patient (often referred to as external beam therapy). Brachytherapy involves the use of sealed radiotherapy sources placed in close proximity to the treated tissue (e.g. intracavitary treatment).

The gray (Gy) is the SI unit of absorbed dose of external beam radiotherapy. It is equivalent to the absorption of one joule of energy per kilogram of absorber. It is also the unit representing the kinetic energy released per unit mass (KERMA) used to measure the absorbed energy for brachytherapy.

Radiotherapy planning, involving three-dimensional localisation of the treatment volume and assessment of the surrounding normal tissue, is a crucial part of the patient's management. This process, called simulation, may result in the use of multiple radiation fields and shielding of normal tissue by lead blocks. Often small tattoos are placed on the patient to aid accurate positioning for each fraction of radiotherapy.

Adverse effects of radiotherapy

Adverse effects occur as either acute toxicity or late radiotherapy damage (Table 7.1).

Acute toxicity results from the loss of surface epithelial cells. Examples of this include the diarrhoea and cystitis commonly experienced by patients receiving radiotherapy to the pelvis, in addition to skin erythema (Figure 7.1; plate 9). Recovery from the acute toxicity usually occurs in a matter of days or weeks following treatment.

Table 7.1 Complications of radiotherapy

Organ/system	Complication
Acute:	
Skin reactions	Erythema and moist desquamation of the skin
Enteritis and colitis	Diarrhoea
Bladder irritability	Frequency and dysuria
Bone marrow suppression	Anaemia, thrombocytopenia, neutropenia
Late:	
Small bowel	Subacute or acute bowel obstruction, bleeding, perforation, fistulae and malabsorption
Large bowel	Proctosigmoiditis, rectovaginal fistula and rectosigmoid obstruction, stricture, perforation or fistulous communication with other intraabdominal organs
Bladder	Contracture with reduced capacity, haemorrhagic cystitis, vesicovaginal fistula, ureteric obstruction and hydronephrosis
Ovarian failure	Menopausal
Vaginal atrophy and stenosis	Sexual problems

Late radiotherapy damage can occur months or even years following treatment. Damage to the bowel or bladder in patients who have received pelvic radiotherapy may occur as a result of progressive vascular changes in small blood vessels. Oedema and fibrosis of the bowel can result in diarrhoea, proctitis and rectal bleeding and, in some cases, in stricture or fistula formation. Late effects on the bladder can result in symptoms of frequency, urgency and, occasionally, haematuria. The use of vaginal dilators and oestrogen (or lubricating creams) should be offered in an attempt to minimise the effects of vaginal shortening and dryness sometimes seen following pelvic radiotherapy. Patients with a medical history of conditions such as inflammatory bowel disease or diabetes are particularly at risk of such complications.

In premenopausal women, even small doses of radiotherapy to the pelvis can cause ovarian failure.

Clinical applications

CERVICAL CANCER

Both surgery and radiotherapy give identical cure rates for patients with early stage cervical cancer. For these women, the aim is to provide the highest cure rate combined with the lowest associated morbidity. In order to decide the most appropriate modality, factors such as the wish for fertility or ovarian preservation with surgery and the possible late sequelae of radiotherapy must be discussed.

Stage Ia tumours are treated with surgery. Stage Ib to stage IIa tumours may be treated with either surgery or radiotherapy. If radiotherapy is preferred, external beam radiotherapy is followed by an intracavitary insertion or two intracavitary insertions followed by external beam to the pelvic sidewalls with central shielding.

Traditionally, radical radiotherapy has been the treatment of choice for stage IIb to stage IVa disease. In addition, for patients following surgery in whom there is lymph node involvement, high-grade disease or close/involved excision margins, adjuvant radiotherapy is recommended. Recently, however, the results of five randomised controlled trials have shown an overall survival advantage for cisplatin-based therapy given concurrently with radiotherapy.[1-3] Although the trials varied in the stage of disease treated, primary or adjuvant treatment setting, dose of radiation and schedule of cisplatin and radiotherapy, they all showed significant survival benefit for the combined approach. Such a combined approach should now be considered for the patient groups outlined above.

There is also a role for radiotherapy (and possibly chemoradiation) in patients who develop pelvic recurrence of their tumours.

ENDOMETRIAL CANCER

Primary radiotherapy is used for those patients unfit for surgery. Although inferior to surgery, it has a 60% five-year survival for stage I disease.

Adjuvant radiotherapy is commonly used for patients with poor prognostic indicators (such as poorly differentiated tumour or deep myometrial involvement). To date, there is no good evidence from randomised controlled trials showing increased survival as a consequence of adjuvant radiotherapy. There is, however, evidence showing a lower rate of vault recurrence in patients who receive adjuvant radiotherapy.[4] The Medical Research Council is currently running the ASTEC trial (A Study in the Treatment of Endometrial Cancer). The trial aims to assess the benefit of adjuvant radiotherapy in patients with high-risk endometrial cancer pathology and no macroscopic disease following surgery. This subject is explored further in Chapter 11.

VULVAL CANCER

Radiotherapy has several potential applications in the management of vulval cancer. For those unfit for surgery, radiotherapy may be the primary treatment modality. More commonly, groin irradiation is used in an adjuvant setting following primary surgery in those with more than one involved groin node or extracapsular spread from one node.[5]

In some patients with extensive tumours, primary surgery could compromise the function of the urethra or anal sphincter. Preoperative treatment with radiotherapy (and chemotherapy in some cases) may shrink the tumour, allowing preservation of function.[6]

Radiotherapy may also be used to treat patients with recurrent vulval cancer in those who either are not fit for surgery or in whom the alternative may be exenterative surgery. For further details on the role of radiotherapy in vulval cancer management, see Chapter 13.

RADIOTHERAPY FOR SYMPTOM CONTROL IN A PALLIATIVE CONTEXT

Radiotherapy is widely used in the management of pain from bone metastases. Short courses of radiotherapy (usually one or two fractions) may also be given to provide haemostasis in patients bleeding from inoperable tumour masses in the vaginal vault. For further details of palliation, see Chapter 15.

SUMMARY

- Radiotherapy: direct and indirect effects of radiation upon cells.
- Four parameters form the basis of radiobiology: repair, reoxygenation, repopulation and redistribution.
- Teletherapy: distant source.
- Brachytherapy: source in close proximity.
- Complications may be early due to acute toxicity or late due to late radiotherapy damage.
- Previous surgery or medical conditions such as diabetes increase the risk of complications.
- Equal cure rates for radiotherapy and surgery in early stage cervical cancer.
- A survival advantage for chemoradiation over radiotherapy alone in more advanced cervical cancer.
- No increase of survival in endometrial cancer through adjuvant radiotherapy but a decrease of vault recurrence.
- Widely used in vulval cancer as adjuvant treatment.
- Primary treatment in vulval cancer if patient unfit for surgery or to 'shrink' tumour preoperatively.

References

1. Keys HM, Bundy BN, Stehman FB, Muderspach LI, Chafe WE, Suggs CL 3rd, *et al*. Cisplatin, radiation and adjuvant hysterectomy compared with radiation and adjuvant hysterectomy for bulky stage 1b cervical cancer. *N Engl J Med* 1999; **340**: 1154–61.

2. Morris M, Eifel PJ, Lu J, Grigsby PW, Levenback C, Stevens RE, *et al*. Pelvic radiation with concurrent chemotherapy compared with pelvic and para-aortic radiation for high risk cervical cancer. *N Engl J Med* 1999; **340**: 1137–43.

3. Rose PG, Bundy BN, Watkins EB, Thigpen JT, Deppe G, Maiman MA, *et al*. Concurrent cisplatin-based radiotherapy and chemotherapy for locally advanced cervical cancer. *N Engl J Med* 1999; **340**: 1144–53.

4. Aalders J, Abeler V, Kolstad P, Onsrud M. Postoperative external irradiation and prognostic parameters in stage I endometrial carcinoma: clinical and histopathologic study of 540 patients. *Obstet Gynecol* 1980; **56**: 419–27.

5. Thomas G, Dembo A, Bryson SCP, Osborne R, DePetrillo AD. Changing concepts in the management of vulval cancer. *Gynecol Oncol* 1991; **42**: 9–21.

6. Boronow RC, Hickman BT, Reagan MT, Smith RA, Steadham RE, *et al*. Combined therapy as an alternative to exenteration for locally advanced vulvovaginal cancer. II. Results, complications, and dosimetric and surgical considerations. *Am J Clin Oncol* 1987; **10**: 171–81.

8 Chemotherapy: principles and applications

Introduction

Chemotherapy is used in a variety of situations in gynaecological oncology. The best known is in the treatment of gestational trophoblastic disease, where single-agent treatment is highly successful for low-risk cases and multi-agent regimens are used in the treatment of higher-risk cases. Gestational trophoblastic disease is one of the few solid tumours that is regularly cured by chemotherapy alone. It is, however, an uncommon tumour. The most common use in gynaecology is in the treatment of epithelial and non-epithelial ovarian cancers.

Chemotherapy is used in an adjuvant setting (after a primary surgical procedure that may or may not have removed all macroscopic disease), in a 'neoadjuvant' fashion (prior to a surgical procedure) and in relapsed or recurrent disease. In cervical cancer, chemotherapy is usually reserved for selected cases of relapsed disease, although, latterly, it has been employed concurrently with radiotherapy in primary treatment (chemoradiation). This principle is also being applied to selected cases of vulval cancer, although less frequently.

In endometrial cancer, chemotherapy is used to treat advanced or relapsed cases where surgery and or radiotherapy are considered

---

USES OF CHEMOTHERAPY IN GYNAECOLOGICAL ONCOLOGY
- Adjuvant and neoadjuvant treatment in ovarian cancer
- Primary treatment of gestational trophoblastic disease
- Relapsed ovarian cancer
- Advanced or relapsed cervical cancer
- Chemoradiation in cervical and vulval cancer
- Advanced and relapsed endometrial cancer
- Sarcomas and non-epithelial ovarian tumours

---

inappropriate, although hormone treatment is also used in these situations. Finally, chemotherapy may be used as sole or part therapy for gynaecological sarcomas. It should be stressed that the evidence supporting the use of chemotherapy in advanced endometrial cancers, sarcomas and some non-epithelial tumours is weak. This is largely a result of the infrequency with which these conditions are encountered.

Treatment intent

In some situations, the intent of treatment may be curative, an example being trophoblastic tumours, while in others the intent is palliative, for example in recurrent epithelial ovarian cancer. It is one of the most basic principles of cancer care that this intent should be clearly understood at the outset. This is not only because clear and understandable patient information requires it but also because without understanding intent it is impossible to balance risks with benefit. Most, if not all, cytotoxic drugs have adverse effects, some of which can be severe and life threatening. These risks may be acceptable to the patient (and her carers) if the benefit is potential cure; they may not be if palliation is the primary objective (see Chapter 15).

Toxicity

In all of the situations above, conventional chemotherapy used to kill tumour cells will also kill normal, healthy cells. This gives rise to treatment-related toxicity such as myelosuppression, emesis, alopecia and peripheral neuropathy. A balance must be achieved between the effect upon tumour cells and the potential morbidity due to treatment-specific toxicities. Some toxic effects of chemotherapy, such as emesis, can be controlled effectively by the use of 5-HT antagonists such as ondansetron, while others, such as severe myelosuppression, can be life threatening.

Drugs with differing toxicities are often used in combination to try to maximise the cytotoxic effect upon the tumour without an associated increase in morbidity.

Many features combine to allow the selection of appropriate agents, toxicity being one important parameter. The objective is of course to choose the least toxic regimen (single agent or combined) that has known activity in the disease. The mechanism of action of various drugs differs, as do their pharmacokinetic properties. In most instances when chemotherapy fails, it is due to the development of drug resistance and thus the prevention of resistance is high on the agenda when treatment is being planned. Strategies to try to prevent the development of drug resistance include the use of non-crossreacting agents in multi-drug regimens, drugs with different toxicities, dose, route of administration and

Table 8.1 Complications of chemotherapy

Organ/system	Complication
Haematological	Myelosuppression, common with carboplatin, can cause granulocytopenia Granulocytopenia: predisposes to sepsis. Use prophylactic, broad-spectrum antibiotics in febrile granulocytopenic patients Thrombocytopenia: with a risk of spontaneous haemorrhage Anaemia: usually presents after several courses of chemotherapy
Gastrointestinal	Nausea and vomiting, common adverse effects. 5-HT_3 antagonists are effective treatment Mucositis: mouth and pharyngeal ulceration Oesophagitis, causing dysphagia, bowel ulceration resulting in diarrhoea or necrotising enterocolitis (NEC) in severe cases with granulocytopenia. Treatment is with intravenous hydration, electrolyte replacement, antimotility drugs e.g. codeine phosphate and vancomycin in NEC
Genitourinary	Acute renal failure: cisplatin, in particular, causes dose-related renal tubular toxicity. Pre- and post-treatment intravenous hydration is used Haemorrhagic cystitis: due to the irritant effect on the bladder mucosa of acrolein, the toxic metabolite of cyclophosphamide. Hydration, diuresis and mesna (sodium mercaptoethane sulfonate) help to prevent this
Hepatotoxicity	Elevation of liver enzymes may occur
Neurotoxicity	Many cytotoxics cause some central or peripheral neurotoxicity Cisplatin produces ototoxicity, peripheral neuropathy, and, rarely, retrobulbar neuritis and blindness Paclitaxel associated with peripheral sensory neuropathy. Neurotoxicity increased with combination cisplatin therapy
Immunosuppression	Suppression of cellular and humoral immunity predispose to opportunistic infection
Hypersensitivity reactions	Associated with carboplatin, paclitaxel and anaphylaxis with cisplatin
Alopecia	Usually reversible, common with paclitaxel; associated with significant psychological morbidity
Gonadal dysfunction	Infertility: many cytotoxics cause infertility. Successful pregnancies have been achieved after cisplatin-based chemotherapy Teratogenicity: all cytotoxics carry the risk of teratogenicity
Second malignancies	Cisplatin is associated with the development of acute leukaemia

dose scheduling to maximise the pharmacokinetic properties of the drugs. Despite these efforts, recurrence and relapse are often seen in the treatment of solid tumours, gynaecological cancers included.

The complications of chemotherapy are described in Table 8.1.

Epithelial ovarian cancer

See also Chapter 10, Ovarian Cancer Standards of Care.

Almost 75% of patients with ovarian cancer have advanced disease at presentation. In this situation, surgery alone is not curative. A large meta-analysis of studies involving almost 7000 patients with ovarian cancer found that cytoreductive surgery had only a small effect on the survival of women with advanced ovarian cancer; the type of chemotherapy was found to be more important.[1] Around 70% of patients exhibit a response to chemotherapy administered in the adjuvant situation. However, only modest improvements in survival are observed for most patients with advanced ovarian cancer, and the overall five-year survival has remained poor, at around 25%, for the last 30 years.[2] Chemotherapy in ovarian cancer is platinum-based and, to date, the addition of newer chemotherapeutic agents has resulted in only modest increases in survival.

During the 1980s, cyclophosphamide and cisplatinum given in combination became first-line therapy. Cyclophosphamide is an alkylating agent, which acts by cross-linkage of DNA. Cisplatinum, developed in the 1960s, has a similar mode of action to the alkylating agents. The adverse effects of cisplatinum include nephrotoxicity, emesis, neurotoxicity and ototoxicicty (Table 7.1).

Carboplatin is an analogue of cisplatinum. It is less nephro- and neurotoxic and causes less vomiting than cisplatinum. Following studies showing comparable activity to cisplatinum, carboplatin was used in the International Collaboration on Ovarian Neoplasms (ICON 2) trial as a single agent versus a combination of cyclophosphamide, doxorubicin and cisplatinum (CAP). There was no difference in outcome between the two groups.[3]

Paclitaxel, one of the taxane group of drugs, was introduced as a first-line therapy in combination with carboplatin. Extracted from the bark of the Western Yew (*Taxus brevifolia*), it acts by stabilising cell microtubules and thus interferes with cell replication. It can cause severe hypersensitivity reactions and its adverse effects include alopecia, neutropenia, myalgia and peripheral neuropathy. The National Institute for Clinical Excellence (NICE) now recommends the combination of carboplatin and paclitaxel as first-line adjuvant therapy in epithelial ovarian cancer (see Chapter 9). The third trial by the ICON group (ICON 3) compared paclitaxel plus carboplatin with either carboplatin alone or CAP. Presented at the American Society of Clinical Oncology (ASCO) meeting in 2000, this large trial of more than 2000 patients, showed no difference in the outcome between the two treatment arms.[4] As a result of this trial, the advantage of paclitaxel in combination with carboplatin over a regimen of single-agent carboplatin alone has been questioned.

Current research in chemotherapy for advanced ovarian cancer focuses on:

- development of new drugs and combinations of drugs: the combination of carboplatin and paclitaxel with drugs such as gemcitabine, docetaxel and topotecan to form 'triplet' chemotherapy regimens
- neoadjuvant chemotherapy: conventional chemotherapy given in three to four cycles prior to surgical debulking of advanced ovarian cancer, followed by three or four further cycles
- intraperitoneal chemotherapy: conventional drugs administered into the peritoneal cavity following surgery via peritoneal catheters
- gene therapy: novel therapeutic agents developed against tumour vasculature or targeting tumour cells directly are undergoing clinical trials at present.

EARLY-STAGE OVARIAN CANCER

In contrast to advanced disease, the benefit of adjuvant chemotherapy has been debated in early stage disease. Five-year survival rates of over 90% can be achieved in stage 1 disease. Presented at the European Cancer Conference in October 2001, the ICON 1 and Adjuvant Clinical Trial In Ovarian Neoplasm (ACTION) studies helped to clarify the situation. For stage I tumours with certain high-risk features such as clear cell histology, there is a clear survival advantage in those patients who received adjuvant chemotherapy.

RECURRENT OVARIAN CANCER

In recurrent disease, chemotherapy for ovarian cancer is always palliative. Platinum-based chemotherapy may be given as a second-line treatment. Response rates are closely related to the time from primary treatment to relapse. Response rates vary from 25% (in those relapsing within one year) to 60% for those with a disease-free interval of more than two years.[5] For platinum-resistant disease, oral etoposide shows response rates of around 27% and is currently used in patients following failure of first- or second-line platinum-based regimens.[6]

Cervical cancer

In general terms, until recently, the first-line therapy for cervical cancer was a choice between surgery and radiotherapy for early stage disease, radiotherapy for advanced disease and chemotherapy was used mainly as an adjuvant treatment in certain high-risk situations or in the context of recurrent disease. Chemotherapy with combinations such as bleomycin [B], ifosfamide [I] and cisplatin [P] (BIP regimen) was used. In addition to the nephrotoxicity of cisplatinum, bleomycin can cause pulmonary morbidity, while ifosfamide can cause neurological morbidity.

In an almost unprecedented action, the *New England Journal of Medicine* published on the internet the results of three studies on chemoradiation in cervical cancer in advance of their publication in the journal itself.[7-9] Following this, the National Cancer Institute of the National Institutes for Health in Washington, USA, issued a clinical announcement stating that 'strong consideration' should be given to the incorporation of concurrent cisplatin-based chemotherapy with radiation therapy in women who require radiation therapy for treatment of cervical cancer.

Taken together, the results of five trials involving almost 2000 women with stage I–IV cervical cancer show a 30–50% reduction in the relative risks of relapse or death. These results do, however, appear to come at the price of increased morbidity, such as bowel toxicity, which may require bowel resection and has in some cases resulted in death. The balance between the improved outcome versus increased morbidity is the subject of debate in the UK, although many gynaecological oncology centres have included chemoradiation in their treatment protocols for the management of cervical cancer.

Endometrial cancer

Unlike patients with epithelial ovarian cancer, the majority of those with endometrial cancer present with early stage disease. Treatment for this group is surgical, with total abdominal hysterectomy, bilateral salpingo-oophorectomy, peritoneal washings and pelvic lymphadenectomy forming part of the staging procedure.

Currently, prognostic factors such as tumour grade, depth of myometrial invasion, lymph node involvement and peritoneal cytology are used to determine the need for adjuvant therapy. This takes the form of radiotherapy, either to the vaginal vault or pelvis. There is no evidence that such treatment prolongs survival.

Several chemotherapeutic approaches have been investigated in endometrial cancer in attempts to improve survival.

Progestogen therapy using drugs such as medroxyprogesterone acetate (MPA) and megestrol have shown response rates of up to 30%, but without evidence of increased survival.

Both platinum- and paclitaxel-based drug combinations have shown similar response rates but, again, these have not translated into improved survival.[10,11]

Vulval cancer

Where possible, the management of vulval cancer is usually surgical in the first instance, with adjuvant radiotherapy in situations where the excision margin is incomplete/inadequate on the vulva and/or the inguinal/pelvic lymph nodes are involved (see Chapter 5).

Chemotherapy, using 5-fluorouracil, cisplatin or both, in combination with radiotherapy, has been used in patients unfit for surgery or in those in whom exenterative surgery would have to be performed in order to excise all tumour. Using this approach response rates of 50–90% have been reported. In cases where complete response has been achieved, some authors suggest that surgical excision of the primary tumour site is not necessary.[12]

This approach has led to interest in preoperative treatment for patients with extensive tumours in whom radical primary surgery would be required in order to remove all tumour. By giving chemoradiation pre-operatively, several studies have shown that the need for radical surgery decreases, for example leading to preservation of the anal sphincter and avoiding the necessity for major plastic reconstructive procedures.[13]

Rare tumours

GESTATIONAL TROPHOBLASTIC TUMOURS

Gestational trophoblastic tumours are the malignant gestational trophoblastic diseases, complete and partial hydatidiform mole being preinvasive. Comprising invasive mole, choriocarcinoma and placental site trophoblastic tumours, these tumours are important, since the vast majority of patients with these conditions are curable with chemotherapy. Patients are referred for follow-up to centres in Dundee, Sheffield or London.

Certain indications for chemotherapy have been established. These include:

- choriocarcinoma on histology
- serum β-hCG > 20000 iu/l more than four weeks after evacuation of the uterus
- metastatic disease
- persistent haemorrhage
- static/rising β-hCG following evacuation of the uterus.

If any of these indications exist, then patients are given chemotherapy based upon their level of risk, low or high. The risk category is calculated using a scoring system that takes many factors into account, including the patient's age, the β-hCG level and whether the preceding pregnancy had been molar.

'Low-risk' patients are treated with intramuscular methotrexate with folinic acid rescue.[14] The 'high-risk' group of patients, together with the small number who develop resistance to methotrexate, are treated with an alternating regimen of etoposide [E], methotrexate [M] and actinomycin D [A] – EMA – and cyclophosphamide [C] and vincristine [O]. The EMA-CO regimen can also be augmented with intrathecal methotrexate in patients with cerebral metastases.[15]

SUMMARY

Ovarian cancer
- Adjuvant therapy recommended for high-risk early stage ovarian cancer.
- For advanced disease, poor five-year survival of around 25%.
- Current adjuvant chemotherapy in advanced disease – carboplatin and paclitaxel.
- Response rates in relapsed disease relate to time since last chemotherapy.

Cervical cancer
- Concurrent cisplatin-based chemotherapy should be considered in all patients who require adjuvant radiotherapy.
- Treatment-related morbidity is likely to be higher in this group.

Endometrial cancer
- Progestogen and platinum-based therapies show response rates of up to 30%.
- No evidence that this translates into prolonged survival.

Vulval cancer
- Good responses to 5-fluorouracil-based chemoradiation regimens.
- Preservation of function and avoidance of extended radical procedures possible using chemoradiation.

Gestational trophoblastic tumours
- Follow-up and treatment via centres in Dundee, Sheffield and London.
- Several indications for chemotherapy.
- If indicated, chemotherapy based on 'low- or 'high-risk' scores.
- High cure rates.

Non-epithelial ovarian tumours
- Chemosensitive tumours often associated with high cure rates.
- Always consider fertility-preserving surgery in women of childbearing age.

NON-EPITHELIAL OVARIAN TUMOURS

The malignant non-epithelial tumours comprise mainly sex cord stromal and germ cell tumours. They generally occur in younger women and, although not common, they form an important group of ovarian tumours because, unlike the epithelial ovarian tumours, long-term survival and cure can often be achieved.

Of the sex cord stromal tumours, granulosa cell tumours may require chemotherapy. Combination therapy with bleomycin [B], etoposide [E] and cisplatin [P] (BEP regimen) is active in this situation.[16]

The malignant germ cell tumours include dysgerminomas and a group of non-dysgerminomas that includes endodermal sinus tumours and teratomas. Combination chemotherapy with BEP or cisplatin [P], vinblastine [V] and bleomycin [B] (PVB regimen) allow response rates of around 90% to be achieved.[17,18] It is worth restating the recommendation that in young women of childbearing age the initial laparotomy for an ovarian tumour should consider fertility preservation due to the potentially curable nature of some of the non-epithelial ovarian tumours.

References

1. Hunter RW, Alexander ND, Soutter WP. Meta-analysis of surgery in advanced ovarian carcinoma: is maximum cytoreductive surgery an independent determinant of prognosis? *Am J Obstet Gynecol* 1992; **166**: 504–11.

2. Thomas H. Cancer of the ovary: advances in chemotherapy. *Trends in Urology, Gynaecology and Sexual Health* 1998; **3**: 11–16.

3. International Collaborative Ovarian Neoplasm Study Collaborators. ICON 2: randomised trial of single-agent carboplatin against three-drug combination of CAP (cyclophosphamide, doxorubicin, and cisplatin) in women with ovarian cancer. *Lancet* 1998; **352**: 1571–6.

4. Colombo N. Randomised trial of paclitaxel (PTX) and carboplatin (CBDCA) vs a control arm of carboplatin or CAP (cyclophosphamide, doxorubicin, and cisplatin): the third International Collaborative Ovarian Neoplasm Study (ICON 3). *Proc Am Soc Clin Oncol* 2000; **19**: 379a.

5. Blackledge G, Lawton F, Redman C, Kelly K. Responses of patients in phase II studies of chemotherapy in ovarian cancer: implications for patient treatment and the design of phase II trials. *Br J Cancer* 1989; **59**: 650–3.

6. Rose PG, Bundy BN, Watkins EB, Thigpen JT, Deppe G, Maiman MA, *et al.* Concurrent cisplatin-based radiotherapy and chemotherapy for locally advanced cervical cancer. *N Engl J Med* 1999; **340**: 1144–53.

7. Keys HM, Bundy BN, Stehman FB, Muderspach LI, Chafe WE, Suggs CL 3rd, *et al.* Cisplatin, radiation and adjuvant hysterectomy compared with radiotherapy and adjuvant hysterectomy for bulky stage 1b cervical cancer. *N Engl J Med* 1999; **340**: 1154–61.

8. Morris M, Eifel PJ, Lu J, Grigsby PW, Levenback C, Stevens RE, et al. Pelvic radiation with concurrent chemotherapy compared with pelvic and para-aortic radiation for high-risk cervical cancer. N Engl J Med 1999; **340**: 1137–43.

9. Rose P, Blessing J, Mayer A, Homesley H. Prolonged oral etoposide as second-line therapy in platinum-resistant or platinum-sensitive ovarian carcinoma: a Gynecologic Oncology Group Study. J Clin Oncol 1998; **16**: 405–10.

10. Burke TW, Munkarah A, Kavanagh JJ, Morris M, LevenbackC, Tornos C, et al. Treatment of advance or recurrent endometrial cancer with single agent carboplatin. Gynecol Oncol 1993; **51**: 397–400.

11. Ball HG, Blessing JA, Lentz SS, Mutch DG. A phase II trial of paclitaxel in patients with advanced or recurrent adenocarcinoma of the endometrium: a Gynecologic Oncology Group study. Gynecol Oncol 1996; **62**: 278–81.

12. Cunningham MJ, Goyer RP, Gibbons SK, Kredentser DC, Malfetano JH, Keys H. Primary radiation, cisplatin, and 5-fluorouracil for advanced squamous carcinoma of the vulva. Gynecol Oncol 1997; **66**: 258–61.

13. Montana GS, Thomas GM, Moore DH, Saxer A, Mangan CE, Lentz SS, et al. Preoperative chemo-radiation for carcinoma of the vulva with N2/N3 nodes: a Gynecologic Oncology Group study. Int J Radiat Oncol Biol Phys 2000; **48**: 1007–13.

14. Howie PW. Trophoblastic disease. In: Whitfield CR, editor. Dewhurst's Textbook of Obstetrics and Gynaecology for Postgraduates. 5th ed. London: Blackwell; 1995. p.556–67.

15. Bower M, Newlands ES, Holden L, Short D, Brock C, Rustin GJ, et al. EMA/CO for high-risk gestational trophoblastic tumours: results from a cohort of 272 patients. J Clin Oncol 1997; **15**: 2636–43.

16. Homesley HD, Bundy BN, Hurteau JA, Roth LM. Bleomycin, etoposide, and cisplatin combination chemotherapy of ovarian granulosa cell tumours and other stromal malignancies: a Gynecologic Oncology Group study. Gynecol Oncol 1999; **72**: 131–7.

17. Brewer M, Gershenson DM, Herzog CE, Mitchell MF, Silva EG, Wharton JT. Outcome and reproductive function after chemotherapy for ovarian dysgerminoma. J Clin Oncol 1999; **17**: 2670–75.

18. Mayordomo JI, Paz-Ares L, Rivera F, Lopez-Brea M, Lopez Martin E, Mendiola C, et al. Ovarian and extragonadal malignant germ-cell tumors in females: a single-institution experience with 43 patients. Ann Oncol 1994; **5**: 225–31

9 Standards of care and multidisciplinary care planning

Definitions

A standard signifies a level or degree of quality that is considered proper or acceptable. Quality is a concept that defines, in both quantitative and qualitative terms, the level of care or service provided. Quality therefore has two components, the first is quantitative and measurable, and the second qualitative and associated with value judgements. It is a relative, not an absolute concept. It is multidimensional. It implies consistency over a period of time and not just the occasional good performance. It should be possible to relate quality to specific standards or criteria, set in advance. Therefore, "standard of care" is specific to the time and location. Setting of standards also depends on the structure of the existing healthcare system, the availability of resources and expertise and the demand of the public. It is important to note that practices considered to be acceptable in one place may not be acceptable in other parts of the world.

A question of great practical significance is whether the standards set should be "gold" or "minimum" standards. While it may seem that to achieve the gold standard is ideal, the overall standard and quality of clinical care are likely to be improved for more people if the minimum standard is to be achieved by all. The standards of care in the following four chapters refers to the "state of the art" at the present moment in time, in the UK.

Communication

Effective communication is crucial to good relationships and to ensure that the outcomes of treatment are optimal for the women concerned. Good communication also promotes cooperation, minimises misunderstanding, anger and anxiety, and enhances satisfaction with care. Healthcare professionals must be sensitive to potential problems with communication and individuals who provide clinical care should have training in communication and counselling skills. Clinical staff need to be aware that patients often find it difficult to take in information given during the consultation, especially just after receiving bad news. Women should be given adequate time to reflect and opportunities to discuss treatment options before making decisions.

A variety of studies have shown that over 90% of women with cancer want full and clear information. Provision of information reduces fear and anxiety, allows patients to express preferences about treatment outcomes and options, and may reduce treatment-related problems. Women should always be given sufficient information to enable them to contribute to decision-making if they wish to do so. Many women also want their partners to be given more information, particularly about the effects of treatment on sexual function. At every stage, they, and when appropriate, their partners or relatives, should be offered clear, full and prompt information in both verbal and written form. This should include information about the disease, diagnostic procedures, treatment options and their effects and, as far as possible, a realistic assessment of anticipated outcome. Sexually active patients and their partners should be offered specific information about possible effects on their relationship. Information about sources of social support and practical help should be given to patients and their partners, in appropriate languages.

While it should be assumed that most women want to be kept fully informed the amount and timing of information should be consistent with individual patients' desire for information. All patients should receive both individual support and guidance and well-produced information leaflets. Patients' preference should take precedence over the views of relatives or carers.

The multidisciplinary team

Team working facilitates coordinated care. Patients managed by teams are more likely to be offered appropriate treatments and to receive continuity of care through all stages of the disease. In gynaecological cancer, treatment by specialist teams is likely to improve survival and quality of life. Specialisation at the level of the cancer centre allows women with rare or more challenging cancers to be treated by clinicians who see enough cases to develop the expertise necessary to manage the disease effectively.

Members of the cancer unit team should consist of a lead gynaecologist, a lead pathologist, a radiologist and a nurse with a special interest in gynaecological cancer.

The cancer unit team should work closely via a network based on a cancer centre. This core team should liaise closely with designated lead gynaecologists at cancer unit level. All members of the cancer centre core team should have a special interest in gynaecological cancer. It should consist of at least two gynaecological oncologists, radiotherapy specialist, chemotherapy specialist, radiologist, histopathologist, cytopathologist and clinical nurse specialists. Specialist nurse input should occur early and may be very effective in reducing patients' distress, increasing satisfaction and improving information flow to patients.

The specialist gynaecological oncology team should meet at least weekly to discuss the management of individual patients. There should be joint or parallel clinics involving different disciplines, so that individual patients can be seen and discussed by two or more team members together. The team should maintain close contact with other professionals who are actively involved in supporting the patient or carrying out the management strategy decided by the team. These include general practitioners/primary healthcare team, gynaecologists and pathologists at the cancer unit level, psychiatrist, psychologist or trained counsellor, cancer genetics specialist, social worker and the palliative care team.

Throughout the care of each patient, there should be a named clinician to whom she principally relates. Such arrangements should be explicit and clearly understood by patients and healthcare professionals, including the primary care team. Patients should be given written information about the members of the team involved in their management.

Information and audit

Finally, setting standards is only the beginning of a long process. Like many other processes, the standard setting cycle involves the setting of standards, the implementation of the action required, evaluation of the outcome and new standards set. The standards should be constantly reviewed and raised through clinical audits. The cancer unit and cancer centre teams should keep a similar minimal dataset so that clinical audits can be performed and the standard of care can be compared. They must

---

CLINICAL SERVICE PROVISION ESSENTIAL FEATURES
- Patient centred care.
- Teams work at different levels of specialisation.
- Multidisciplinary teams.
- Effective communication between primary care, cancer units and cancer centres.
- Mutually agreed evidence-based guidelines and policies.
- Regular team meetings.
- Standard improvement through clinical audits.

---

be fully committed to maintaining the quality and have effective mechanisms to deal with those who do not meet the standards.

The cancer unit gynaecology team should meet regularly, at least once a fortnight to discuss the management of individual patients. Decisions should follow documented local clinical policy, which should be decided by the team in collaboration with the specialist gynaecological oncology team at the linked cancer centre. The team should have adequate support to ensure that all decisions are recorded and communicated to patients and their general practitioners.

10 Ovarian cancer standards of care

Current status of screening for ovarian cancer

It is generally recognised that early-stage disease has a better prognosis (see Chapter 1) and there is no doubt that screening can detect cases of ovarian cancer in asymptomatic women and the majority of those cases detected will have early-stage disease. There have been several attempts to use varying combinations of physical examination, TVS and serum CA125 assay to detect these early stages of ovarian cancer. Unfortunately, the modalities currently available are hampered by unacceptable sensitivity and specificity (Table 10.1). Only 50% of patients with stage I disease have raised serum CA125 levels and a significant proportion of healthy women have elevated levels of CA125. Consequently, there are concerns over false positive results, which can lead to unnecessary intervention in healthy women, while, on the other hand, some women with cancer will remain undetected. There are currently three randomised controlled trials underway, whose conclusions are awaited.

CURRENT STANDARD
- A systematic review of up-to-date evidence, including over 100 000 women, suggests that at the current time there is insufficient evidence to support screening of low-risk or high-risk women.[1]

Family history

Whereas women with no family history of ovarian cancer have a 1.5% lifetime risk, those with one affected first-degree relative (mother, daughter, sister) have a 5% risk and women with two first-degree relatives have a 7% risk. The risk is somewhat lower for women with one first-degree and one second-degree relative (grandmother, aunt) with ovarian cancer. Overall, approximately 5–10 % of cases of ovarian cancer are thought to be familial. It has become well established that inherited mutations in either *BRCA 1* or *BRCA 2* confer Mendelian dominant

Table 10.1 Sensitivity and specificities of screening modalities for ovarian cancer

Screening modality	Cut off (u/ml)	Sensitivity (%)	Specificity (%)
CA125 alone	35	72–100	81–98
CA125 alone	65	72–83	93–99
Ultrasound alone		89–100	42–75

genetic predisposition to both breast and ovarian cancer with approximately 80% penetrance. *BRCA 1* is found in 5% of women diagnosed with ovarian cancer before the age of 70 years. Unfortunately, this is a large gene with over 100000 base pairs, any one of which may be mutated. It is only currently possible to screen within families in whom a specific mutation has been identified. Estimates of the lifetime cancer risk associated with *BRCA* mutations are variable and depend upon the population studied, ranging from 15–60% for ovarian cancer. There are likely to be several genes that predispose to ovarian cancer, some associated with colon cancer syndromes such as hereditary non-polyposis colorectal cancer. The genetic predisposition for an individual woman can be difficult to determine without expert knowledge. Multiple primary cancers in one individual or related early-onset cancers in a family tree are suggestive of a predisposing gene. Outwith those families where a specific gene abnormality is identifiable, there are few families in which it is possible to be sure of dominant inheritance, but where four first-degree relatives have early-onset or bilateral breast cancer in combination with ovarian cancer, the risk of inheriting a mutated gene is close to 50%.

Presentation and diagnosis

See also Chapter 4, Presentation, Investigation and Diagnosis.

Since early diagnosis is associated with better prognosis, significant improvements in the cure rate for ovarian cancer are likely to result from prompt diagnosis and referral to suitable specialists. Unfortunately, the symptoms of ovarian cancer are often non-specific and may mimic gastrointestinal conditions, with problems such as bloating, abdominal pain, change of bowel habit, backache and weight loss being prominent. The non-specific nature of the symptoms is associated with a delay in diagnosis of up to one year.[4]

It is estimated that 5–10% of women will undergo a surgical procedure for a suspected ovarian neoplasm during their lifetime and 13–21% of these women will be found to have an ovarian malignancy. Since the majority

CURRENT STANDARD

- The determination of risk for a woman and her family members should prompt referral to a geneticist. However, these referrals should be limited to high-risk women to prevent overwhelming the system.

CRITERIA FOR CATEGORISATION OF A WOMAN AS HIGH-RISK FOR OVARIAN CANCER

- Two or more first-degree relatives affected by ovarian cancer.
- One first-degree relative with ovarian cancer and one with breast cancer diagnosed before the age of 50 years.
- One first-degree relative with ovarian cancer and two with breast cancer diagnosed before the age of 60 years.
- An individual with a mutation of one of the genes known to predispose to ovarian cancer.
- Three first-degree relatives with colorectal cancer with at least one diagnosed below the age of 50 years, as well as one case of ovarian cancer.
- There has been a move towards prophylactic oophorectomy in apparently high-risk women. This has become a popular measure, perhaps in advance of evidence to support its efficacy. It is gratifying, however, that data suggesting up to a 98% risk reduction for high-risk women are beginning to accumulate.[2,3] The standard of care for this group of women at increased genetic risk of cancer is evolving rapidly and continuing research will necessitate refinement of the standards.

of masses are benign, it is important to try to determine preoperatively whether a patient is at high risk of ovarian malignancy, in order to ensure proper management. To determine whether an adnexal mass requires surgery and the appropriate preparation and intervention, preoperative evaluation must include:

- complete history
- examination
- TVS
- serum CA125 levels.

CURRENT STANDARD

- All healthcare workers should be aware of the difficulties in diagnosing ovarian cancer and should retain a high level of suspicion around suggestive symptoms.

The use of a 'risk of malignancy index' may improve the selection of cases that would benefit from referral to a gynaecological oncologist. Studies suggest that a combination of age, level of serum CA125 and ultrasound findings could offer an 80–90% sensitivity and specificity for detecting ovarian cancer.

Surgery

See also Chapter 5, Surgical Principles.

OPTIMAL DEBULKING

There is considerable evidence that volume of disease remaining at the completion of primary surgery is related to patient survival. Various maximum residual disease criteria ranging from 0.5–2.0 cm have been established. Such studies led to the established standard of 'optimal debulking surgery', which aims to reduce the residual disease to the minimum achievable.[5] However, the recommendation is based only on largely retrospective series and is therefore questionable. It is possible that the ability to optimally debulk some women may simply reflect less aggressive tumour biology and thus any apparent improvement in survival may be spurious. A prominent meta-analysis suggests only a modest improvement in median survival for maximally debulked surgery. This benefit was much smaller than the gain drawn from adjuvant chemotherapy with platinum-containing regimens.[6]

CURRENT STANDARD
- Despite these reservations about the quality of the data, the current recommendation is to aim for minimum residual disease, leaving deposits with a maximum individual diameter of 2 cm.

CHOICE OF SURGEON

Observational studies provide convincing evidence that management by a gynaecological oncologist is associated with better survival. These data suggest that three years after treatment by a specialist gynaecologist, a woman's chance of dying from ovarian cancer is 25% lower than if treated by a general gynaecologist and 33% lower than after treatment offered by a general surgeon.[7] In this influential study, the greatest benefit was observed among women with stage III disease. Differential use of platinum chemotherapy did not explain this survival advantage. Specialist gynaecologists more often debulked tumour to less than 2 cm than general gynaecologists in stage III cases (36.3% versus 28.7%, $P = 0.07$).

> **CURRENT STANDARD**
> Ovarian cancer or cases with a high level of suspicion should be managed by a trained gynaecological oncologist.

IMPORTANCE OF COMPLETE STAGING

Correct staging is vital, particularly for women with apparently early-stage disease. On reinvestigation, up to 31% of women with apparently early-stage disease were found to have a more advanced stage of the disease.[8] Women with stage I or II disease as determined by a gynaecological oncologist have a significantly better overall and progression-free survival than those operated on by a generalist, suggesting more thorough staging. Unfortunately, audit results show that many women are not adequately staged and there are marked variations between hospitals. This study suggested that women who were not appropriately managed according to guidelines died sooner.[9]

Washings and omental biopsies should form part of the routine management of a woman with an ovarian cyst at any age. These simple procedures allow for adequate staging, which is particularly important when determining the subsequent management of a woman who might want to retain her fertility. Adequately assessed stage I disease treated by unilateral salpingo-oophorectomy is associated with an excellent prognosis that may not be worse than pelvic clearance.

The role of lymph node sampling is more contentious. According to FIGO staging, lymph node status is required and it is not infrequent for positive nodes to be found even in early-stage disease (Table 10.2). There is, however, no convincing evidence to show that such sampling actually improves outcome for women with stage I or II disease.

Table 10.2   Incidence of positive nodes per stage of ovarian cancer

Stage	Incidence (%)
I	≤ 24
II	50
III	74
IV	73

CURRENT STANDARD
- Adequate staging should, as a minimum, include peritoneal washings (or assessment of ascites) and an omental biopsy, as well as removal of the affected cyst and/or ovary.

BORDERLINE TUMOURS

A subcategory of serous tumours is recognised that may be separated from clearly benign and clearly malignant tumours. The behaviour of these tumours is more indolent but they may nevertheless be associated with extraovarian disease of similar histology. Thus, it is possible to have advanced-stage borderline disease. The terminology has led to much confusion regarding the natural history of the category. Other terms such as 'carcinoma of low-malignant potential' or 'atypical proliferating tumour' have been suggested and may be easier to conceptualise. However, the term 'borderline' is accepted by the World Health Organization and will remain for the foreseeable future. Patients with borderline tumours tend to be younger than patients with frank malignancies and overall prognosis is good, but recurrences have been reported as late as 20 years after initial presentation. A woman with a borderline tumour diagnosed after a unilateral salpingo-oophorectomy may be advised that the recurrence risk without further surgery is approximately 7%.

CURRENT STANDARD
There is no evidence that treatment of borderline tumours with adjuvant chemotherapy is beneficial.

A particular challenge is posed by the group of women who have serous borderline tumours that exhibit invasive omental or peritoneal implants. In a study of 44 women with serous borderline tumours, four women with invasive implants died of their disease between three and nine years, despite chemotherapy.[10]

Chemotherapy

See also Chapter 8, Chemotherapy: Principles and Applications.

STAGE I DISEASE

Approximately 25% of women with newly diagnosed ovarian cancer present with stage I disease (Figures 10.1; plate 9: Figure 10.2; plate 10). Although the outcome for this group is relatively good, a significant proportion of these women die from their malignancies. Much attention has been focused on identifying the subsets of women at highest risk of relapse who may benefit from adjuvant therapy. There is currently no published evidence from randomised controlled trials to clearly support adjuvant chemotherapy in early-stage disease other than in an as yet unclearly defined group with high-risk prognostic factors. The importance of cyst rupture as a prognostic feature may have been overstated previously.

CURRENT STANDARD
- The role of adjuvant chemotherapy in stage I disease is currently under review following the presentation of data from the ICON I and ACTION studies, which suggest a benefit for adjuvant chemotherapy.[11]

ADVANCED DISEASE

Platinum-based chemotherapy improves survival among women with ovarian cancer beyond stage I (Figure 10.3; plate 10). Data from a meta-analysis of trials involving over 5500 women in 37 randomised controlled trials show that chemotherapy including platinum (excluding taxanes) improved survival rates at five years by 5% from 25–30%.[12] In 1998, ICON 2, a large ovarian cancer study involving over 1500 women, showed that there was no difference in survival comparing carboplatin against the traditional three-drug combination of CAP (cyclophosphamide, doxorubicin and cisplatin). The single agent was significantly less toxic.

Several trials have assessed the role of combinations of platinum with paclitaxel. In the Gynaecological Oncology Group (GOG) trial 111, the cisplatin and paclitaxel was judged to be superior to the platinum-based control arm, with an improvement of overall response rate, median progression-free interval and overall median survival.[13] These favourable data were confirmed by a European-Canadian Intergroup trial (OV10).[14] In contrast, in a further GOG trial (GOG 132) there was no difference in survival between cisplatin alone and the combination of paclitaxel with cisplatin. The ICON 3 study has released European data on the first and only trial comparing paclitaxel plus carboplatin against carboplatin alone or a (non-taxane) carboplatin-based control arm. ICON 3 found no significant difference in survival with combination therapy. The results of ICON 3, in accordance with the GOG 132 study, appear to contradict the earlier positive results seen with taxane/platinum combinations. NICE has so far supported the use of taxane/platinum combinations. The guidance, which has been made available to the NHS in England and Wales, recommends that the drug paclitaxel should be used to treat women with ovarian cancer as a standard initial therapy.

CURRENT STANDARD
- Combination chemotherapy involving a taxane and a platinum should be offered for advanced ovarian cancer. In patients who may not be able to tolerate this combination, carboplatin alone can be effective.

Role of interval debulking surgery

In the event of being unable to achieve primary optimal debulking, there has been a move towards interval debulking surgery. In this protocol, women receive half of their planned cycle of chemotherapy and are then offered a further attempt at debulking. The evidence in support of this practice is currently limited. A European trial involving over 300 women suggested a 33% reduction in risk of death following interval debulking surgery (95% CI 10–50) and a significant progression-free and overall survival ($P = 0.01$).[15] A smaller study showed a two-year survival rate of 15% in those not undergoing a second procedure and 30% for those undergoing interval debulking surgery. This was not statistically significant. The standard of care in this situation is currently undefined.

Role of second-look laparotomies

Second-look laparotomies have been considered after completion of chemotherapy. There are no data to show that therapeutic decisions based upon results of this procedure alter outcomes for the patient.

CURRENT STANDARD
Second-look laparotomies should not be undertaken as part of routine management.

Role of radiotherapy

There does not appear to be a role for radiotherapy in the adjuvant setting but there may be a role in palliation in recurrent disease. This area lacks randomised controlled data.

> **CURRENT STANDARD**
> There is no evidence to support the use of adjuvant radiotherapy in epithelial ovarian cancer.

Follow-up

The serum CA125 level is a useful marker of disease recurrence and thus worth measuring in follow-up in those women whose level was raised at the time of initial diagnosis. The significance of serum CA125 levels before treatment is uncertain but it does significantly correlate with survival when measured one month after the third course of chemotherapy for patients with stage III and IV disease. If CA125 levels normalise after treatment, a subsequent rise is associated with active disease but the utility of treatment before symptoms is currently unclear and is the subject of a continuing trial.

The ideal and most effective follow-up of asymptomatic women who have completed primary debulking surgery and chemotherapy and have no clinical evidence of disease is unclear. Optimal intervals have not been determined. Current practice is to follow up every three to four months in the first two years and to reduce that to six-monthly intervals until five years have elapsed.

A combination of serum CA125 level and general physical and pelvic examination has been shown to detect progression of disease in 90% of patients. Radiological examination such as CT scan has not been shown to improve the detection of recurrence.

Management of patients with relapsed disease

Most patients (approximately 75%) respond to initial therapy but it is a sad fact that over 55% will relapse within two years. For the overwhelming majority of patients who relapse, the salvage therapy currently available for ovarian cancer is not curative. Therefore, the goals of follow-up and treatment need to incorporate quality-of-life considerations as an integral part of the treatment. Patients who have relapsed after primary chemotherapy with platinum can be divided into two groups based on the interval to relapse. Patients who relapse within six months have a poor prognosis and poor response to platinum-containing regimens. Those who relapse after six months have a higher likelihood of response to platinum-containing regimens. Depending on the duration of the treatment-free interval (i.e. the length of time between the last dose of first-line therapy and the planned initiation of second-line treatment), the anticipated objective response rate is predicted to range from 20% to as high as 70%. Response rates nearly equivalent to that of primary chemotherapy may be achieved when the treatment-free interval exceeds 24 months.

There is a lack of randomised trials to determine the optimal therapy for recurrent disease. ICON 4 is addressing this deficit by currently comparing platinum with platinum/paclitaxel for women who relapse at least six months after prior treatment with platinum. For platinum resistant or refractory women, recent NICE guidance supports the use of topotecan as second-line therapy. When a patient relapses for a second time, there is almost no possibility of cure. Temporary response rates of 15% have been reported with a variety of therapeutic agents.

CURRENT STANDARD
- Current best practice is to offer further combination platinum and paclitaxel therapy to platinum sensitive women. It has a median overall response rate of 35% but it is unclear if this significantly prolongs survival.

THE ROLE OF SURGERY IN RELAPSED DISEASE

Retrospective data would suggest that surgery to resect isolated recurrences may be beneficial for patients in good general condition with a relatively long interval since prior chemotherapy. However, this benefit is only likely to extend to small subset of highly selected patients. These include patients with a long disease-free survival (greater than two years) who had optimal primary debulking surgery. Surgery may, however, be important for palliation, such as for the treatment of bowel obstruction in a patient whose quality of life stands to benefit from this intervention.

NON-EPITHELIAL OVARIAN NEOPLASMS

The relative rarity of this group of cancers results in a relative paucity of data upon which to determine management. The above recommendations about adequate surgery and debulking still apply. The relatively early age of presentation of germ cell tumours necessitates conservative surgery in the majority.

References

1. Bell R, Petticrew M, Luengo S, Sheldon TA. Screening for ovarian cancer: a systematic review. *Health Technol Assess* 1998; **2**: 1–84.

2. Eisen A, Rebbeck TR, Wood WC, Weber BL. Prophylactic surgery in women with a hereditary predisposition to breast and ovarian cancer. *J Clin Oncol* 2000; **18**: 1980–95.

3. Weber BL, Punzalan C, Eisen A, Lynch HT, Narod SA, Garber JE, *et al*. Ovarian cancer risk reduction after bilateral prophylactic oophorectomy (BPO) in BRCA1 and BRCA2 mutation carriers (abstract). *Am J Hum Genet* 2000; **67** Suppl 2. [www.faseb.org/genetics/ashg00/f251.htm]. Accessed 24 September 2003.

4. Flam F, Einhorn N, Sjovall K. Symptomatology of ovarian cancer. *Eur J Obstet Gynecol Reprod Biol* 1988; **27**: 53–7.

5. Hoskins WJ. Epithelial ovarian carcinoma: principles of primary surgery. *Gynecol Oncol* 1994; **55**: S91–S96.

6. Hunter RW, Alexander ND, Soutter WP. Meta-analysis of surgery in advanced ovarian carcinoma: is maximum cytoreductive surgery an independent determinant of prognosis? *Am J Obstet Gynecol* 1992; **166**: 504–11.

7. Junor EJ, Hole DJ, Gillis CR. Management of ovarian cancer: referral to a multidisciplinary team matters. *Br J Cancer* 1994; **70**: 363–70.

8. Young RC, Decker DG, Wharton JT, Piver MS, Sindelar WF, Edwards BK, *et al*. Staging laparotomy in early ovarian cancer. *JAMA* 1983; **250**: 3072–6.

9. Wolfe CD, Tilling K, Raju KS. Management and survival of ovarian cancer patients in south east England. *Eur J Cancer* 1997; **33**: 1835–40.

10. de Nictolis M, Montironi R, Tommasoni S, Carinelli S, Ojeda B, Matias-Guiu X, *et al*. Serous borderline tumors of the ovary. A clinicopathologic, immunohistochemical, and quantitative study of 44 cases. *Cancer* 1992; **70**: 152–60.

11. Vergote I, Trimbos BJ, Guthrie D, Parmar MK, Bolis G, Mangioni C, *et al*. Results of a randomised trial in patients with high-risk early ovarian cancer, comparing adjuvant chemotherapy with no further treatment following surgery. In: American Society of Clinical Oncology. *2001 Annual Meeting Summaries*. Alexandria, VA; 2001. p. 802.

12. Aabo K, Adams M, Adnitt P, Alberts DS, Athanazziou A, Barley V, *et al*. Chemotherapy in advanced ovarian cancer: four systematic meta-analyses of individual patient data from 37 randomized trials. Advanced Ovarian Cancer Trialists' Group. *Br J Cancer* 1998; **78**: 1479–87.

13. McGuire WP, Hoskins WJ, Brady MF, Kucera PR, Partridge EE, Look KY, *et al*. Cyclophosphamide and cisplatin compared with paclitaxel and cisplatin in patients with stage III and stage IV ovarian cancer. *N Engl J Med* 1996; **334**: 1–6.

14. Piccart MJ, Bertelsen K, James K, Cassidy J, Mangioni C, Simonsen E, *et al*. Randomized intergroup trial of cisplatin-paclitaxel versus cisplatin-cyclophosphamide in women with advanced epithelial ovarian cancer: three-year results. *J Natl Cancer Inst* 2000; **92**: 699–708.

15. Van der Burg ME, van Lent M, Buyse M, Kobierska A, Colombo N, Favalli G, *et al*. The effect of debulking surgery after induction chemotherapy on the prognosis in advanced epithelial ovarian cancer. Gynecological Cancer Cooperative Group of the European Organization for Research and Treatment of Cancer. *N Engl J Med* 1995; **332**: 629–34.

11 Endometrial cancer standards of care

Introduction

The subsequent discussion will follow the order of patient journey from originally attending their general practitioners, referral to secondary care to care in cancer centres and palliative care services.

Primary to secondary care

Women presenting with postmenopausal bleeding are at risk of having endometrial cancer and investigations to confirm or exclude such a possibility should be performed (see also Chapter 4). As the risk of having cancer is approximately 10%, these women should be referred for gynaecological assessment at a local cancer unit, where there is a gynaecologist with special interest in gynaecological oncology.

Many women with postmenopausal bleeding will not require an urgent assessment, but they should be given an early appointment. Those at increased risk of cancer should be seen within two weeks of their general practitioner's referral.

CURRENT STANDARD
- Indication for urgent referral (to be seen within two weeks):
  - more than one or a single heavy episode of postmenopausal bleeding in a woman over 55 years old and not on hormone replacement therapy (HRT)
  - unexpected or prolonged bleeding lasting more than four weeks after stopping HRT.

- Indication for an early appointment (usually within four weeks):
  - any postmenopausal bleeding (not covered above)
  - unscheduled bleeding on HRT.

Diagnosis and investigations

CONFIRMING CANCER

See also Chapter 4, Presentation, Investigation and Diagnosis.

After referral, transvaginal ultrasound should be performed to assess the thickness of the endometrium. TVS is a safe, cost-effective method for excluding endometrial cancer. It is highly reliable for detection of endometrial cancer. For women with postmenopausal vaginal bleeding, it has a negative predictive value approaching 100% in terms of excluding endometrial cancer. TVS therefore allows over 75% of women to be reassured immediately. Many invasive procedures can be avoided. It is also safe to manage women expectantly after negative transvaginal ultrasound and cervical cytology.[1,2]

Endometrial biopsy should be carried out if the endometrium thickness is 5 mm or greater. A range of sampling devices can be used and they appear to be equally accurate, giving a correct diagnosis of cancer in over 80% of cases.[3,4] The Pipelle aspirator is normally used because it causes less pain and has better patient acceptability than other devices, such as the Novak, the Vabra and the Karman curette. Diagnostic hysteroscopy and dilatation and curettage should be used only when outpatient biopsy is unsuccessful or with persistent abnormal bleeding. Outpatient hysteroscopy is available in some centres and is an alternative to inpatient hysteroscopy in situations where endometrial biopsy fails to either confirm or refute the diagnosis.

ASSESSING DISEASE EXTENT

In order to optimise the choice of treatment, preoperative evaluation is essential with respect to pathology of a biopsy and radiological assessment of the extent of disease. The risk of lymph node involvement, and thus the stage of the cancer, are closely correlated with the depth of myometrial invasion and the tumour grade. Apart from measuring the endometrial thickness, TVS should also assess the depth of myometrial invasion. It has a sensitivity of 66–86% and a specificity of 83–90% to detect tumour invasion extending through more than half of the myometrium.[5–7] MRI is also valuable in assessing the degree of myometrial penetration (see below). Tumour grade can be assessed by pathological examination of biopsy samples. These two findings help selection of women with good prognosis to be treated safely in local hospitals.[8] Women with stage Ia or Ib, grade 1 or 2 disease (about 40% of cases) should have their treatment at the cancer unit. Women who are judged to have more advanced or higher-risk cancers (stage Ic; stage I, grade 3 or higher and those with

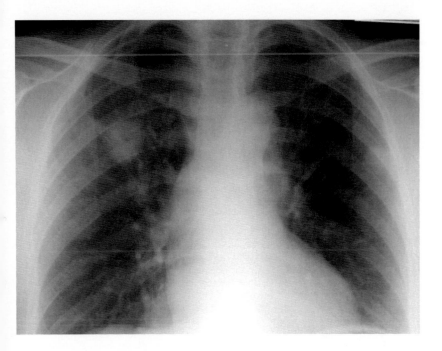

Figure 11.1 Pulmonary metastases in endometrial cancer

morphological or other features associated with poor prognosis) should be referred to cancer centres. The waiting time from diagnosis to treatment ideally should not exceed one month.

All patients with confirmed disease should have a chest X-ray to exclude pulmonary metastases (Figure 11.1). MRI should be available for pretreatment staging at the cancer centres. MRI is more sensitive than ultrasound or CT for assessing myometrial invasion (Figure 11.2) and tumour spread beyond the uterus but its cost-effectiveness is unclear.[9]

Surgical treatment and staging of disease

See also Chapter 5, Surgical principles.

Women with endometrial cancer should be treated by surgery whenever possible. This is because stage for stage, women treated with surgery have a better prognosis than women who are treated with radiotherapy alone.[10–12] Most women with endometrial cancer can be treated by surgery alone, with minimal morbidity and high survival rates (over 75% at five years in major European centres). The standard procedure is total abdominal hysterectomy and bilateral salpingo-oophorectomy with or

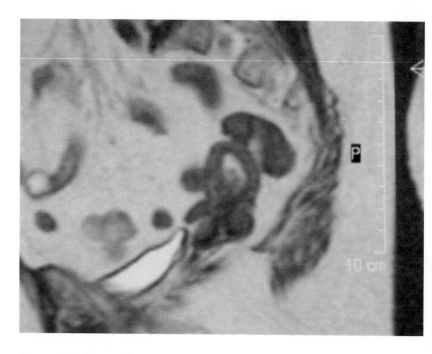

Figure 11.2 Magnetic resonance image showing intrauterine mass and fluid

without retroperitoneal lymph node dissection.

The current standard staging criteria for endometrial cancer were established by the FIGO in 1988 (see Appendix 1). Although this is a surgical staging system, there is no systematic staging schema. The operative staging of women with endometrial cancer usually consists of peritoneal washing, hysterectomy and adenectomy with visualisation and palpation of intra-abdominal, retroperitoneal and pelvic organs or surfaces. Biopsies of suspicious abnormalities often serve as the primary and only method of additional intraoperative staging.

Ideally, knowledge of the presence or absence of lymph node involvement through lymphadenectomy rather than indirect risk assessment by tumour grade and myometrial invasion should define the need for adjuvant radiotherapy (Figure 11.3: plate 11). Prospective evaluation of intraoperative interpretation suggests that surgical impression of nodal involvement is inaccurate, even in experienced hands.[13] Lymphadenectomy can be performed safely, without significant added morbidity, when performed by a trained and experienced gynaecological oncologist.[14,15] The presence of a gynaecological oncologist is also associated with a 25-fold increase in the chance of complete surgical staging.[14,16]

Routine lymphadenectomy is not performed in the UK, as many patients are treated by general gynaecologists who may not have the surgical skills. Moreover, many patients are medically unfit or obese, limiting the scope for extensive surgery; and many patients have early disease, which does not justify lymphadenectomy. In the absence of clinically apparent extrauterine disease, careful postoperative histological evaluation of the specimens is undertaken to assess the risk of extrauterine disease and the need for adjuvant radiation therapy for women deemed at high risk of recurrence.

Adequate exposure is an absolute essential for surgical staging. This is best performed through a midline vertical incision, which allows full evaluation of the abdomen, permitting adequate inspection of the upper abdomen, pelvic and para-aortic nodes, and allows omental biopsy if required. Laparoscopic surgery has been advocated as an alternative approach to treatment of women with endometrial cancer, with less morbidity.[17] Complete surgical staging including lymph node dissection can be accomplished. However, laparoscopic staging is performed in relatively few institutions and there are few data on the feasibility of the procedure among most centres. Importantly, there exists a relatively long learning curve of 50 to 100 cases to master the techniques. Moreover, long-term results after laparoscopic surgery have not been reported.

Radiotherapy and chemotherapy

See also Chapter 6, Radiotherapy: principles and applications and Chapter 8, Chemotherapy: principles and applications.

Women with endometrial cancer should be treated by surgery whenever possible. Primary radiotherapy may be used to treat those with advanced disease for whom surgery is considered inappropriate, or when surgery is contraindicated. Five-year survival rates after radiotherapy alone are around 40%. Radiotherapy should also be offered to women with locally recurrent endometrial cancer who have not already had pelvic radiotherapy.

There is wide variability between centres in the use of adjuvant radiotherapy and no consensus on which patients should receive this type of treatment or on the type of radiotherapy (external beam, vault brachytherapy or both) that should be given. There is currently no reliable research evidence on which decisions may be based. When the status of the lymph nodes is unknown, it is common to refer patients with high-grade tumours, deep myometrial invasion and tumour extension into the cervix for postoperative external radiotherapy. The rationale is to reduce the risk of locoregional recurrence. A prospective randomised study of more than 700 patients with apparent stage I endometrial cancers failed to show a survival benefit of postoperative adjuvant external radiotherapy.[18]

COMMON INDICATIONS FOR POST-HYSTERECTOMY ADJUVANT RADIOTHERAPY
- tumour grade: grade 2 and 3 tumours
- myometrial invasion: greater than 50% penetration
- cervical involvement
- poor histological variants: clear cell and papillary serous
- positive pelvic lymph nodes.

Radiotherapy can have lasting adverse effects, including damage to the vagina, bowel and urinary tract. The combination of radiotherapy and surgery (particularly lymphadenectomy) may cause lymphoedema of the legs and lower abdomen. Apart from improved pelvic control, this study also reported a four-fold increase in treatment-related morbidity after pelvic radiation.[18] Although the risk of local recurrence was higher in women treated with surgery alone, management of recurrent disease in those not having received radiotherapy resulted in excellent survival. Delivery of external radiotherapy in patients with apparent stage I endometrial cancer adds to cost and morbidity without a documented increase in survival or favourable effect on quality of life.[18]

Many gynaecological oncologists have questioned the benefit of postoperative adjuvant radiotherapy in those patients who have been surgically staged and found to be node negative, as no survival benefit has been demonstrated. There is growing evidence that survival in this group of patients is excellent without the incorporation of postoperative radiotherapy. The overall risk of recurrence is less than 10%. Disease-related deaths are often associated with failure to control recurrent distal disease, which in most instances is not related to pelvic disease control.

No evidence has been identified to suggest that primary chemotherapy is beneficial as an adjuvant for women with endometrial cancer. Systemic chemotherapy has typically been reserved for women with disseminated primary disease or extrapelvic recurrence. There is no standard regimen. Treatment should be considered palliative rather than curative. Although multi-drug regimens generally produce higher response rates than single agents, response duration is generally brief. This needs to be balanced against the significant and more severe adverse effects of combined therapy than single agent therapy.[19]

A meta-analysis of the results of seven randomised controlled trials has shown that adjuvant progestogen therapy confers no survival benefit.[20]

Progestogens should not be used for adjuvant treatment for endometrial cancer. The role of oestrogen replacement remains controversial. In early-stage disease, there is probably no increased risk of relapse and therefore oestrogen containment could be considered in selected cases.

Palliative treatment and care

As with any cancer, women with advanced endometrial cancer, whether in hospital or in the community, should have access to specialist palliative care on a 24-hour basis and there should be local arrangements to ensure continuity of care. The aim of palliative care is to maintain and improve quality of life and the whole person should always be considered. It is important to provide both optimum relief from symptoms and to maintain their social and psychological wellbeing. Particular attention should be given to adequate pain control, for which effective interventions should be readily available.

A variety of interventions, ranging from surgery to supportive care, may be necessary to improve quality of life for women going through the late stages of cancer. Patients and their relatives should be given realistic information about potential benefits, limitations and adverse effects of interventions and their views should always be respected.

Most women with advancing cancer are likely to wish to remain at home for much of the duration of their illness. Patients should be helped to remain in the place they prefer, whether this is their home, hospital or hospice and should whenever possible be allowed to choose where they wish to die.

Palliative aspects of care are addressed in more detail in Chapter 15.

Post-treatment support and follow-up

At present, there is no evidence to support routine follow-up for women whose cancer is in remission. However, these women are likely to need aftercare and support during the recovery following primary treatment and should have continuing access to appropriate services.

Care following primary treatment aims to identify and manage physical and psychological morbidity following primary treatment and to detect recurrent disease and initiate treatment as early as possible. Women should be informed about specific problems that may develop some time after treatment.

Patient-centred care

Delay between initial suspicion of cancer and treatment, and particularly between initial assessment at local hospitals and referral to specialist centres, should be kept to a minimum. Women's anxiety increases with increasing time between suspicion of cancer and the beginning of treatment. For 30% of women with endometrial cancer, there are delays of six months or more between the onset of symptoms and the beginning of treatment. This may mean that the cancer develops to a higher stage. However, there is no evidence that survival is impaired by delays of up to three months. Nevertheless, reducing delay will reduce women's anxiety and may permit earlier treatment. This can be achieved by the establishment of rapid assessment services for women with postmenopausal bleeding.

Organisation and provision of services

The optimum management of endometrial cancers requires close coordination between the primary healthcare team, the treatment teams at both cancer unit and cancer centre levels, the palliative care team and patients and their families. Effective communication is essential between all care settings. Decisions about management should follow local clinical policy, which should be demonstrably evidence-based. All members of teams should be involved in discussions on local policy decisions and auditing adherence to them. Teams should be jointly responsible for audit and participation in clinical trials.

For endometrial cancer, the cancer unit should provide a rapid and appropriate assessment service at the local level for women presenting with postmenopausal bleeding. The designated lead gynaecologist should normally carry out surgery for early (Stage Ia or Ib, grade 1 or 2) cancers of the endometrium. Specialist support from a cancer centre should be available, if needed. Women with late-stage endometrial cancers should be referred to the cancer centre following initial assessment at the cancer unit, since these are relatively uncommon and may present particular challenges. It is crucial to have mutually agreed criteria for rapid referral and effective channels of communication between primary care, cancer units and cancer centres.

References

1. Gull B, Carlsson S, Karlsson B, Ylostalo P, Milsom I, Granberg S. Transvaginal ultrasonography of the endometrium in women with postmenopausal bleeding: is it always necessary to perform an endometrial biopsy? *Am J Obstet Gynecol* 2000; **182**: 509–15.

2. Ferrazzi E, Torri V, Trio D, Zannoni E, Filiberto S, Dordoni D. Sonographic endometrial thickness: a useful test to predict atrophy in patients with postmenopausal bleeding. An Italian multicenter study. *Ultrasound Obstet Gynecol* 1996; **7**: 315–21.

3. Stovall TG, Solomon SK, Ling FW. Endometrial sampling prior to hysterectomy. *Obstet Gynecol* 1989; **73**: 405–9.

4. Dijkhuizen FP, Mol BW, Brolmann HA, Heintz AP. The accuracy of endometrial sampling in the diagnosis of patients with endometrial carcinoma and hyperplasia: a meta-analysis. *Cancer* 2000; **89**: 1765–72.

5. Szantho A, Szabo I, Csapo ZS, Balega J, Demeter A, Papp Z. Assessment of myometrial and cervical invasion of endometrial cancer by transvaginal sonography. *Eur J Gynaecol Oncol* 2001; **22**: 209–12.

6. Arko D, Takac I. High frequency transvaginal ultrasonography in preoperative assessment of myometrial invasion in endometrial cancer. *J Ultrasound Med* 2000; **19**: 639–43.

7. Olaya FJ, Dualde D, Garcia E, Vidal P, Labrador T, Martinez F, *et al.* Transvaginal sonography in endometrial carcinoma: preoperative assessment of the depth of myometrial invasion in 50 cases. *Eur J Radiol* 1998; **26**: 274–9.

8. Frei KA, Kinkel K, Bonel HM, Lu Y, Zaloudek C, Hricak H. Prediction of deep myometrial invasion in patients with endometrial cancer: clinical utility of contrast-enhanced MR imaging: a meta-analysis and Bayesian analysis. *Radiology* 2000; **216**: 444–9.

9. Kinkel K, Kaji K, Yu KK, Segal MR, Lu Y, Powell CB, *et al.* Radiologic staging in patients with endometrial cancer: a meta-analysis. *Radiology* 1999; **212**: 711–18.

10. Surwit EA, Joelsson I, Einhorn N. Adjuvant radiation therapy in the management of stage I cancer of the endometrium. *Obstet Gynecol* 1981; **58**: 590–5.

11. Grigsby PW, Perez CA, Camel HM, Kao MS, Galakatos AE. Stage II carcinoma of the endometrium: results of therapy and prognostic factors. *Int J Radiat Oncol Biol Phys* 1985; **11**: 1915–23.

12. Hernandez W, Nolan JF, Morrow CP, Jernstrom PH. Stage II endometrial carcinoma: two modalities of treatment. *Am J Obstet Gynecol* 1978; **131**: 171–5.

13. Arango HA, Hoffman MS, Roberts WS, DeCesare SL, Fiorica JV, Drake J. Accuracy of lymph node palpation to determine need for lymphadenectomy in gynaecologic malignancies. *Obstet Gynecol* 2000; **95**: 553–6.

14. Orr JW, Roland PY, Leichter D, Orr PF. Endometrial cancer: is surgical staging necessary? *Curr Opin Oncol* 2001; **13**: 408–12.

15. Podratz K, Mariani A, Webb M. Staging and therapeutic value of lymphadenectomy in endometrial cancer. *Gynecol Oncol* 1998; **70**: 163–4.

16. Orr JW, Roland PY, Orr PJ, Bolen DD, Hutcheson SL. Subspecialty training: does it affect the outcome of women treated for a gynaecologic malignancy? *Curr Opin Obstet Gynecol* 2001; **13**: 1–8.

17. Eltabbakh GH, Shamonki MI, Moody JM, Garafano LL. Laparoscopy as the primary modality for the treatment of women with endometrial carcinoma. *Cancer* 2001; **15**: 378–87.

18. Creutzberg CL, van Putten WL, Koper PC, Lybeert ML, Jobsen JJ, Warlam-Rodenhuis CC, *et al.* Surgery and postoperative radiotherapy versus surgery alone for patients with Stage I endometrial carcinoma: multicenter randomised trial. *Lancet* 2000; **355**: 1404–11.

19. Burke TW, Gershenson DM. Chemotherapy as adjuvant and salvage treatment in women with endometrial carcinoma. *Clin Obstet Gynecol* 1996; **39**: 716–27.

20. Martin-Hirsch PL, Lilford RJ, Jarvis GJ. Adjuvant progestagen therapy for the treatment of endometrial cancer: review and meta-analyses of published randomised controlled trials. *Eur J Obstet Gynecol Reprod Biol* 1996; **65**: 201–7.

12 Cervical cancer standards of care

Introduction

Many of the downward changes in the mortality trend for cervical cancer described in Chapter 1 are attributable to behavioural trends and to the introduction of the NHS Cervical Screening Programme. However, it is hoped that in achieving high standards of care for those patients diagnosed with cervical cancer a further impact can be made. It is also hoped that this will bring improvements in patients' quality of life, irrespective of whether or not they are curable, from the pretreatment stage and throughout their treatment regimen and the post-treatment period.

Presentation

See also Chapter 4, Presentation, Investigation and Diagnosis.

Women with early stage disease may not have symptoms and may be detected through the cervical screening programme. While a cervical smear cannot diagnose an invasive process, as it is an investigation of cytological abnormality, it can suggest this if highly atypical cells are seen, often in association with debris from the tumour. Even in those women where the cervical smear report is suggestive of a preinvasive lesion, there still remains the possibility that the lesion may be cancerous. Careful colposcopy will pick up many of these lesions and in the remainder the diagnosis will be made by histopathological assessment.[1] Any woman who has a smear suggestive of invasion, high-grade CIN or AIS should be referred and seen at a colposcopy clinic within four weeks. It is essential to be aware that a recent negative cervical smear does not exclude malignancy, as a necrotic tumour may not desquamate abnormal cells. Similarly, an abnormal appearance or texture of the cervix may raise the suspicion of malignancy and indicates referral for further investigation irrespective of the cervical smear report.

In clinically detected lesions, symptoms are usually present and include:

- postcoital bleeding
- intermenstrual bleeding
- postmenopausal bleeding
- offensive bloodstained vaginal discharge.

Comprehensive treatment guidelines and quality standards for cervical screening and the management of abnormal smears have been published by the Cervical Screening Programme (see Chapter 4).

CURRENT STANDARD
- A clinically suspicious cervix should prompt referral.
- A negative cervical smear does not exclude cancer.
- Smears suggestive of malignancy or high-grade CIN should be referred within four weeks.

Diagnosis and staging

A patient presenting to her general practitioner with intermenstrual bleeding or persistent vaginal discharge, or whose cervix looks or feels abnormal, should be referred to a gynaecologist. If there is a high index of suspicion that a malignancy is present, she should be referred to the gynaecological assessment service at a cancer unit rather than to a general gynaecologist and obstetrician. Diagnosis is based upon a biopsy. If the lesion is large and clinically highly suspicious, then a directed biopsy will often suffice. In smaller lesions and especially in microscopic cancer (Stage Ia), the whole lesion should be included in the biopsy in order to allow for accurate histological substaging. This will most likely require either a cone biopsy or a large loop or laser excision. If invasive disease is confirmed at histology a specialist pathologist at a cancer centre should also review the specimen in order to check the accuracy of staging.

Subsequent management depends on the stage of the disease (see Appendix 1). If the specimen obtained at large loop excision of the transformation zone (LLETZ) or cone biopsy shows no evidence of tumour at the margins and it falls within the measurement parameters of stage Ia disease, these patients may be managed at cancer unit level by the lead oncology gynaecologist. If clinical or histological examination at the unit level suggests a higher stage of disease, the patient should be referred to the specialist gynaecological team within a cancer centre. Staging of cervical cancer is covered in detail in Chapter 4.

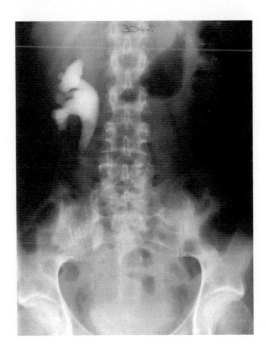

Figure 12.1 Hydronephrosis demonstrated on intravenous urogram

Other investigations

Cancer centres should have MRI facilities available and MRI should be included in the preoperative work-up of the patient, although it will not affect the clinical staging of the disease. Some centres are replacing the intravenous urogram (Figure 12.1) with transvaginal ultrasound, as it is effective in detecting hydroureter and hydronephrosis.

It is essential that staging is performed in an accurate and systematic manner in order to maximise the chances of a patient receiving the most appropriate management. In the UK, it is hoped that the development of cancer networks will lead to an improvement in the adequacy of staging, which previously has been shown to be less than ideal. An audit of cervical cancer during the 1989–93 period revealed that a large proportion of patients were not correctly staged initially; 58% of women with higher than stage Ia disease had no X-ray performed preoperatively, 47% had no FIGO staging described in their notes and around 10% had inappropriate conservative surgery and subsequently required salvage surgery or radiotherapy.[2] It has also been shown that the type of hospital in which the staging is undertaken affects the staging adequacy. Teaching hospitals, with oncology support, have a higher adequacy of staging rate compared with non-teaching hospitals, without oncology support.[3] The obvious concern is that inadequate staging could lead to under-treatment, with potentially disastrous consequences and overstaging could lead to unnecessary morbidity associated with therapy.

Although the disease is staged clinically, there is an increasing use of imaging techniques. The use of MRI scanning is increasing and has been shown to be superior to CT scanning and clinical examination in terms of determining extent of tumour. It is also the optimal test for determining lymph node status when compared with CT scan[4] and is as effective as lymphangiography while being less invasive, making it a more acceptable option where available.[5]

CURRENT STANDARD
- Large biopsies including the whole lesion are required to accurately substage stage Ia disease.
- MRI and ultrasound are useful adjuncts to clinical staging.
- Accurate staging is an essential prerequisite to good treatment planning.
- Stage Ia disease can be managed in cancer units.

Treatment of cervical cancer

STAGE IA CERVICAL CANCER

Surgery is appropriate for the majority of women with stage Ia cervical cancer (see also Chapter 5). For very early disease, i.e. stage Ia1, where the depth of invasion is less than 3 mm, the incidence of positive lymph nodes is around 1% (negligible if less than 1 mm) and so for the majority of women local excision with LLETZ or cone biopsy is likely to be sufficient. Obviously, this decision has to be made with the informed consent of the patient. When the depth of invasion is 3–5 mm, the risk of positive lymph nodes increases to around 4%. The incidence of node positivity in stage Ia2 disease has been variably reported and lymphadenectomy should be considered, probably in those who show evidence of lymph-vascular invasion. In cases of Ia disease, local excision is usually sufficient to achieve local control. Thus, fertility can be spared in those women who wish to retain it. There is no evidence to support the use of radical surgery in stage Ia disease.

STAGE IB AND IIA CERVICAL CANCER

The currently available evidence would suggest that surgery (see also Chapter 5) and radiotherapy (see also Chapter 7) are equally effective in

CURRENT STANDARD

- Local excision is sufficient treatment for stage Ia1 disease.
- Stage Ia2 disease can also be managed by local excision, lymphadenectomy may be required for extensive lymphovascular space involvement although the incidence of nodal disease is still low.
- Fertility sparing is possible in all stage Ia disease.
- As parametrial involvement is not reported in stage Ia disease, radical surgery is not necessary.

the treatment of stage Ib cervical cancer. It is possible, although as yet not proven, that chemoradiation may offer improved outcomes. Surgery and radiotherapy have different morbidity profiles that will usually have the major influence on decision making. As with stage Ia disease, women with small Ib tumours (usually stage Ib1 tumours) may have scope to retain their fertility. This group of women may be offered treatment by lymphadenectomy with trachelectomy, a procedure that has been reported to result in successful pregnancies.[6] This is a crucial area for decision making by the patient and her partner and should only be undertaken after close liaison with the gynaecological oncology team in the cancer centre setting.

For patients who do not wish to retain their fertility and for whom local excision has been an inadequate surgical treatment, the choice lies between radical hysterectomy with pelvic lymphadenectomy or radical radiotherapy. Both are equally effective in terms of outcome. Radical surgery should be carried out by specialist gynaecological oncologists working in cancer centres. It has been shown that radicality of surgery is appropriately greater when patients are treated in specialist centres and that the five-year survival of these patients is increased.[3,7] Surgery alone should be offered whenever possible, since it is less likely to result in impaired sexual enjoyment, bowel or bladder function.

If the patient is not fit to undergo surgery or she elects to be treated by radiotherapy, she should be offered radiotherapy. Most centres would now consider chemoradiation as the optimal form of treatment. For early-stage cervical disease, this has been shown to be as effective in terms of survival.[8-11] Radiotherapy carries the risk of radiation-associated morbidity, including diarrhoea, cystitis and tiredness during or soon after the treatment and an 8% risk of long-term adverse affects, including problems with the bladder, bowel and vagina. Pelvic radiotherapy in younger women may also precipitate menopause and lead to infertility.

Adjuvant radiotherapy is widely used after radical surgery to reduce the risk of recurrence in women with positive nodes. Although it has been shown in several retrospective studies that adjuvant radiotherapy reduces the risk of recurrences within the pelvis, there is no firm evidence that it increases long-term survival.[12,13]

Radical radiotherapy should be offered when surgery is unlikely to remove the tumour completely or when the risk of requiring postoperative radiation is considered high. This will help to reduce the number of cases where surgery and radiotherapy are employed as this has been shown to be associated with even higher levels of morbidity. A clinical oncologist with a specialist interest in gynaecological oncology should administer radiotherapy and chemoradiation. This is usually given in the form of intracavitary brachytherapy and external beam radiotherapy. The question of whether to give extended field radiotherapy (i.e. beyond the pelvic nodes) has been addressed in a number of studies.[14,15] Overall, there does not seem to be a significant benefit from extended field irradiation for all cases, as there is a significant increase in radiotherapy-related morbidity. However, it may prove to be appropriate in cases of proven para-aortic node involvement.

CURRENT STANDARD
- Surgery and radiotherapy are equally effective in terms of survival. Choice of therapy will depend on morbidity and patient choice.
- Radical trachelectomy with lymphadenectomy allows scope for fertility sparing in some women who have small (Ib1) tumours.
- Members of the multidisciplinary team who have special expertise in the disease should give radical surgery and radiotherapy in gynaecological cancer centres.
- No benefit has been demonstrated from the use of extended field radiation.

LOCALLY ADVANCED CERVICAL CANCER (STAGE IIB AND ABOVE)

These cases do not usually lend themselves to primary surgical management. Treatment is based on radiotherapy and chemotherapy. A significant development in the management of cervical cancer has occurred in the last three years. Several randomised controlled trials have shown that concurrent platinum-based chemotherapy given with radiotherapy significantly improves survival and progression-free survival among women with disease ranging from stage Ib-IVa when compared with the use of radiotherapy without chemotherapy.[16–19] The majority of centres in the UK now use a regimen of chemoradiation for these patients and an increasing number of these centres are also using chemotherapy for those patients receiving adjuvant radiotherapy where nodal disease is present in patients who have undergone radical surgery. While the results of these studies showed the efficacy of cisplatin in this setting, there is a gradual move towards the use of carboplatin in the UK.

CURRENT STANDARD
- Primary management is based on radiotherapy.
- Chemoradiation may be superior to radiotherapy alone, albeit with higher morbidity.
- Radiation with concurrent platinum is the combination of choice.

EXENTERATIVE SURGERY

For those patients with extensive cancer confined to the central pelvis (recurrent cancer of the cervix or extensive primary disease), exenterative surgery can be considered if the patient is suitably fit and understands the risks and likely outcomes associated with such extensive surgery. Where the patients are carefully selected and the surgery is performed by highly skilled surgeons, a five-year survival rate has been reported.[20-23] The surgical morbidity associated with this surgery is around 2–4%. In the three reporting studies above, a common finding was a zero percent survival rate (between one and five years) in those patients found to be node-positive. This level of surgery should only be undertaken in cancer centres and only by those surgeons who are performing this type of surgery on a regular basis. It is essential that careful preoperative counselling is given to these patients, as they will have to undergo diversion of the urinary and/or gastrointestinal tracts and this is likely to have a major impact on their psychological, social and sexual function. Patients should then receive counselling from an appropriately trained and informed member of the multidisciplinary oncology team, typically the consultant performing the surgery and one of the nurse specialists from the team.

CURRENT STANDARD
- Exenterative surgery is highly specialised and should be performed only by expert teams in cancer centres.
- Patients with positive lymph nodes do not benefit from this type of surgery.
- Patients should be carefully counselled with regard to the risks and morbidity of this type of surgery.

Post-treatment support and follow-up

There is no reliable evidence on which to base recommendations for routine follow-up of asymptomatic women after treatment for cervical cancer. In the majority of cancer centres in the UK, patients are followed up for five years and then discharged if all is well. No evidence supports the use of cervical cytology in follow-up and this practice should be discouraged.

There is one possible role for cytology in follow up. This is when there is a high index of suspicion of residual VAIN. For this reason, all patients undergoing surgery for cervical cancer should first have the vaginal vault assessed colposcopically in order to determine if the atypical transformation zone involves the vagina.

Treatment for all gynaecological cancers can result in physical, psychosocial and sexual morbidity. In the immediate postoperative period, the patient should, through local policy, receive help, support and appropriate treatment without delay, if it is required. They should be informed of specific problems that may develop some time after treatment for cervical cancer such as lymphoedema, bowel or bladder dysfunction and should have clear routes for access to appropriate specialist help if signs or symptoms appear. This will depend upon close liaison between cancer centres and units, general practitioners and supporting nursing care. These are principles that apply to all the gynaecological cancers.

CURRENT STANDARD
- Although there are no data to support the regular use of routine follow-up in treated patients, it may be of value in the early detection of recurrence, late morbidity and in providing psychological support for patients.
- The routine use of cervical cytology should be restricted to those in whom there is a high degree of suspicion that they may develop VAIN.

Management of patients with recurrent disease

One of the objectives of follow-up is to detect recurrent disease. Although many believe that the early detection of recurrence will positively influence the outcome of subsequent therapy, no data exist to support this.

Disease may relapse centrally, in the pelvis, at the pelvic sidewall or by widespread and distant metastases. Adjuvant radiation is often given after primary surgery to reduce the risk of central pelvic relapse. If patients have received primary radiotherapy as their sole treatment, detecting pelvic relapse may be difficult, as it is not always easy to distinguish postradiation fibrosis from recurrence. If doubt persists after imaging, Trucut® biopsies may be required to confirm recurrence.

CENTRAL PELVIC RELAPSE

This may present with dull central pelvic pain, bleeding or discharge. There may be alterations in either bowel or bladder function. The condition may be asymptomatic. If the central pelvic disease remains mobile, exenteration may be a treatment option. If the disease is fixed and the patient has not been treated previously by radiotherapy, this would be the first choice of treatment. Most centres would probably consider chemoradiation if the patient were fit, although none of the published data on chemoradiation specifically addresses the issue of relapsed disease.

PELVIC SIDEWALL RECURRENCE

The symptoms associated with recurrence on the sidewall may relate to nerve root involvement (groin and leg pain), lymphatic occlusion (lymphoedema in the affected limb), ureteric compression (usually asymptomatic) or visceral pain. A fixed mass palpable on the sidewall in association with confirmatory imaging is usually considered diagnostic, although Trucut® or image-guided biopsies may be required. These cases are not amenable to further surgery and definitive treatment is by radiation, if not previously treated. In previously irradiated patients, treatment will usually be palliative in the form of pain control and/or chemotherapy. The results of chemotherapy are disappointing in previously irradiated tumours.

CURRENT STANDARD
- Mobile central pelvic recurrence can be managed by pelvic exenteration in selected patients.
- In previously non-irradiated patients, central pelvic and sidewall recurrence should be managed by radiotherapy.
- Although chemoradiation is considered in relapsed patients, no data are as yet available to show that this is superior to radiotherapy alone.
- Bone metastases are best managed by radiotherapy.
- Chemotherapy may have a role in the treatment of soft tissue metastases that are not in previously irradiated sites.

DISTANT METASTASES

The presentation varies with the site and type of metastasis. Bone metastases will usually present with pain and can be well controlled by radiotherapy. Soft tissue metastases will usually be considered for chemotherapy and reasonable response rates have been recorded in previously non-irradiated tissues. There are few long-term survivors in patients with recurrent carcinoma of the cervix.

References

1. Shafi MI. Cervical cancer In: Shafi MI, Luesley DM, Jordan JA, editors. *Handbook of Gynaecological Oncology*. London: Churchill Livingstone; 2000.

2. Jackson S, Murdoch J, Howe K, Bedford C, Sanders T, Prentice A. The management of cervical carcinoma within the south west region of England. *Br J Obstet Gynaecol* 1997; **104**: 140–44.

3. Wolfe CD, Tilling K, Bourne HM, Raju KS. Variations in the screening history and appropriateness of management of cervical cancer in South East England. *Eur J Cancer* 1996; **32A**: 1198–204.

4. Patrick J, Winder E, editors. *Cervical Screening: A Practical Guide for Health Authorities*. Publication No. 7. Sheffield: NHSCSP; 1997.

5. NHS Cervical Screening Programme. *Quality Assurance Guidelines for the Cervical Screening Programme*. Report of a Working Party. Sheffield: NHSCSP; 1996.

6. Kim SH, Choi BI, Lee HP, Kang SB, Choi YM, Han MC, *et al*. Uterine cervical cancer: comparison of CT and MR findings. *Radiology* 1990; **175**: 45–51.

7. Scheidler J, Hricak H, Yu KK, Subak L, Segal MR. Radiological evaluation of lymph node metastases in patients with cervical cancer. A meta-analysis. *JAMA* 1997; **278**: 1096–101.

8. Shepherd JH, Crawford RAF, Oram DH. Radical trachelectomy: a way to preserve fertility in the treatment of early cervical cancer. *Br J Obstet Gynaecol* 1998; **105**: 912–6.

9. Bissett D, Lamont DW, Nwabineli NJ, Brodie MM, Symonds RP. The treatment of stage 1 carcinoma of the cervix in the west of Scotland 1980–1987. *Br J Obstet Gynaecol* 1994; **101**: 615–20.

10. Landoni F, Maneo A, Colombo A, Placa F, Milani R, Perego P, *et al*. Randomised study of radical surgery versus radiotherapy for stage Ib-IIa cervical cancer. *Lancet* 1997; **350**: 535–40.

11. Morley GW, Seski JC. Radical pelvic surgery versus radiation therapy for stage I carcinoma of the cervix (exclusive of microinvasion). *Am J Obstet Gynecol* 1976; **126**: 785–98.

12. Newton M. Radical hysterectomy or radiotherapy for stage I cervical cancer. A prospective comparison with 5 and 10 year follow-up. *Am J Obstet Gynecol* 1975; **123**: 535–42.

13. Soisson AP, Soper JT, Clarke-Pearson P, Berchuck A, Montana G, Creasman WT. Adjuvant radiotherapy following radical hysterectomy for patients with stage Ib and IIa cervical cancer. *Gynecol Oncol* 1990; **37**: 390–5.

14. Kinney WK, Alvarez RD, Reid GC, Schray MF, Soong SJ, Morley GW, *et al*. Value of adjuvant whole pelvis irradiation after Wertheim hysterectomy for early stage squamous carcinoma of the cervix with pelvic nodal metastasis: a matched-control study. *Gynecol Oncol* 1989; **34**: 258–62.

15. Rotman M, Pajak TF, Choi K Clery M, Marcial V, Grigsby PW, *et al*. Prophylactic extended-field irradiation of para-aortic lymph-nodes in stage IIb and bulky Ib and IIa cervical carcinomas. Ten-year treatment results of RTOG 79-20. *JAMA* 1995; **274**: 387–93.

16 Haie C, Pejovic MH, Gerbaulet A, Horiot JC, Pourquier H, Delouche J, *et al*. Is prophylactic para-aortic irradiation worthwhile in the treatment of advanced cervical cancer? Results of a controlled clinical trial of the EORTC radiotherapy group. *Radiother Oncol* 1998; **11**: 101–2.

17. Rose PG, Bundy BN, Watkins EB, Thigpen JT, Deppe G, Maiman MA, *et al*. Concurrent cisplatin-based radiotherapy and chemotherapy for locally advanced cervical cancer. *N Engl J Med* 1999; **340**: 1144–53.

18. Keys HM, Bundy BN, Stehman FB, Muderspach LI, Chafe WE, Suggs CL 3rd, *et al*. Cisplatin, radiation and adjuvant hysterectomy compared with radiation and adjuvant hysterectomy for bulky stage Ib cervical carcinoma. *N Engl J Med* 1999; **340**: 1154–61.

19. Morris M, Eifel PJ, Lu J, Grigsby PW, Levenback C, Stevens RE, *et al*. Pelvic radiation with concurrent chemotherapy compared with pelvic and para-aortic radiation for high-risk cervical cancer. *N Engl J Med* 1999; **340**: 1137–43.

20. Whitney CW, Sause W, Bundy BN, Malfetano JH, Hannigan EV, Fowler WC Jr, *et al*. Randomized comparison of fluorouracil plus cisplatin versus hydroxyurea as an adjunct to radiation therapy in stages IIb–IVa carcinoma of the cervix with negative para-aortic lymph nodes: a Gynecologic Oncology Group and Southwest Oncology Study Group. *J Clin Oncol* 1999; **17**: 1339–48.

21. Robertson G, Lopes A, Beynon G, Malfetano JH, Hannigan EV, Fowler WC Jr, *et al*. Pelvic exenteration: a review of the. Gateshead experience 1974–92. *Br J Obstet Gynaecol* 1994; **101**: 529–31.

22. Shepherd JH, Ngan HS, Neven P, Fryatt I, Woodhouse CR, Hendry WF, *et al*. Multivariate analysis of factors affecting survival in pelvic exenteration. *Int J Gynecol Cancer* 1994; **4**: 361–70.

23. Morley GW, Hopkins MP, Lindenauer SM, Roberts JA. Pelvic exenteration, University of Michigan: 100 patients at 5 years. *Obstet Gynecol* 1989; **73**: 934–43.

13 Vulval cancer standards of care

Introduction

The rarity of vulval cancer (see Chapter 1) has meant that few if any robust randomised trials have been performed. Evidence has been based largely on personal series and are therefore always subject to the risk of selection bias. Centralisation of care should go some way to allow properly designed trials to be conducted and there are data that also suggest that this may result in an improved outcome.[1,2,3]

> **CURRENT STANDARD**
> - Vulval cancer should be managed in cancer centres by multidisciplinary teams.

When considering standards of care in any disease situation, one of the primary areas to address is prevention: whether there is a preventative strategy that can be assessed in quality terms.

Prevention and predisposing conditions

There is no screening strategy to either prevent the development of invasive cancer or detect disease at an early and asymptomatic stage. In approximately one-third of cases there will be evidence of a pre-existing HPV-related disorder (VIN)[4,5] and an additional one-third may have evidence of a vulval maturation disorder. The aetiology is far from clear however and it is more than likely that there is more than one putative oncogenic process (see Chapter 1).

Women with Paget's disease of the vulva are not only at higher risk of having occult invasion at the time of diagnosis but may also be at a higher risk than women with VIN of developing cancer in the future.[6] Melanoma *in situ* is also felt to be associated with a higher risk.[7,8]

An important point is that of follow-up in these at-risk conditions. It would seem to be impractical to offer regular follow-up to all women with lichen sclerosus even though there is a 4% (approximate) lifetime risk of developing cancer.[9] Similarly, low-grade VIN is associated with a very low rate of progression to cancer and may not warrant follow-up. Current practice is to keep high-grade VIN, Paget's disease and melanoma-*in situ* on annual review at least. Other potential predisposing conditions are discharged from follow-up having been counselled with regard to the level of risk. They are also informed of the changes in signs and symptoms that may accompany malignant transformation. Their primary carers are also given this information and asked to review the woman annually.

CURRENT STANDARD
- There is no screening test for vulval cancer.
- Women with predisposing conditions should be counselled with regard to risk.
- Where risk is considered to be high, review should be arranged.

Primary detection and referral

"Everyone with suspected cancer will be able to see a specialist within two weeks of their GP deciding that they need to be seen urgently and requesting an appointment." This is the core statement underpinning the Government statement on cancer care in the NHS. The gynaecological guidelines were introduced in October 2000.

Primary carers are being asked to make decisions on risk of cancer based upon:

- sociodemographic (age, gender)
- relevant risk factors (smoking, family history)
- symptoms
- findings on clinical examination
- results of investigation (primary care).

However, this has to be put in perspective as symptom profiles, in particular, vary in incidence depending on the baseline population. Given the population incidence of vulval cancer, there will be approximately 0.03 cases per 2000 population; thus, in ten years, an average general practitioner will see three cases. Simple, accurate guidance for primary carers is therefore essential.

GUIDELINES FOR REFERRAL FROM PRIMARY CARE

Although the disease can be asymptomatic, pain, itching, burning and soreness are the most frequent symptoms and almost 90% of women will admit to some symptoms. All symptomatic postmenopausal women and all premenopausal women not responding to simple first-line therapy should be examined. Genital warts are common but less so in the elderly and should prompt early biopsy if not responding to simple topical therapies. Other features to look for include:

- a swelling, polyp or lump
- an ulcer
- colour changes (whitening, pigment loss or gain)
- elevation and or irregularity of surface contour
- a clinical 'wart'
- irregular fungating mass
- an ulcer with raised, rolled edges
- enlarged groin nodes.

Ninety percent of all vulval cancers will have an easily visible lesion at the time of first presentation.

CURRENT STANDARD
- All women with vulval symptoms should have the vulva examined.
- Any area of suspicious epithelium should prompt a gynaecological referral.
- Warts not responding to primary therapy should be biopsied.

Making the diagnosis

See also Chapter 4, Presentation, Investigation and Diagnosis.

The diagnosis is based on biopsy. Several scenarios may present themselves.

1. There is a large, fungating or ulcerated mass, which clinically is malignant. This lesion is unlikely to be resectable without causing significant morbidity and should therefore be biopsied and not completely resected. The biopsy should be taken from the edge of the lesion so as to include adjacent, macroscopically normal epithelium (Figure 13.1: plate 11). This procedure can be performed under local anaesthesia, thus avoiding additional general anaesthesia, particularly in elderly frail women.

2. There is a small, well-circumscribed mass that is suspicious for malignancy. In this situation, a diagnostic biopsy may be taken as already detailed or a wide local excision can be performed if this will

not be unduly morbid or compromise function. If an excisional biopsy is planned, this should be radical and should ensure a minimum clearance of 1 cm at least on all margins, including the deep margin (Figure 13.2; plate 12). As the site of the lesion on the vulva may have a bearing on future therapy, this should be recorded, preferably by photography, prior to its excision. For excisional biopsies therefore:
› record the site of the lesion (photography)
› record the size of the lesion (macroscopic and pathologic)
› aim for clearance margins of at least 1cm and clearance of 1 cm on depth as well.

3. The final situation occurs when a lesion, not thought to be cancer, is biopsied. In this scenario, re-excision may be necessary as part of treatment. Exceptions might include lesions with superficial invasion only (see below).

BIOPSY INFORMATION

Reporting standards in oncology are now becoming standardised. As management of many cancers is highly dependent upon histopathological confirmation and characteristics it is easy to understand the importance of this. In vulval cancer the report on the biopsy should include reference to the following:

- Is it cancer?
- What histological type?
- Depth of invasion?
- Clearance margins?
- Associated epithelial abnormalities?
- Involvement of capillary-like spaces?

Histological subtypes

Knowledge of the subtype is important, as it may influence the need for lymph node dissection. All squamous cancers, with the exception of verrucous and basal cell carcinomas, have a risk of lymph node spread. The only exceptions here are those cancers with less than 1 mm depth of invasion (as measured from the base of the nearest adjacent papilla). This group (superficially invasive or stage Ia vulval cancer) is associated with less than 1% lymph node metastasis and the current consensus is that nodal resection is not required.

Malignant melanoma is also considered as a situation where lymphadenectomy is not indicated, as long as there is no evidence to suggest macroscopically involved nodes. The overwhelming prognostic determinant in this disease is the depth of invasion (Clark's level) and not node status as it is in squamous disease. Prophylactic lymphadenectomy has not been shown to have independent prognostic significance in melanoma although some authorities feel that resection of bulky involved nodes may influence the course of the disease and at the least confer some palliative benefit.

CURRENT STANDARD
- Diagnosis is based upon a representative biopsy or biopsies from the most atypical areas.
- Diagnostic biopsies should include normal adjacent epithelium.
- Excisional biopsies should only be considered in small lesions where a wide margin of normal tissue can also be excised.

Planning treatment

Once the diagnosis has been confirmed, treatment options need to be considered. The major factors that influence treatment planning are:

- the need to address the possibility of nodal involvement
- the extent of disease
- the patient's suitability for treatment.

It may be necessary to consider additional investigations such as imaging to assess nodal status and distant metastases. There may be a need to consider additional biopsies or fine-needle aspirates from enlarged nodes. It should be remembered, however, that currently clinical assessment of groin lymph nodes is notoriously inaccurate and that imaging techniques to evaluate lymph nodes are still in the phase of clinical enquiry and not clinical practice.

NODAL STATUS

Although the frequency with which lymph nodes are involved in squamous and adenocarcinomas varies, the potential for nodal disease should be addressed in all but certain subtypes and in stage Ia disease.

Currently, approximately 30% of all operated vulval cancers will have involved lymph nodes and the outcome relates closely to nodal status (Figure 13.3).

Furthermore, the type of nodal involvement will influence outcome and subsequent adjuvant therapy. If nodes are found to contain only microscopic disease, then adjuvant groin irradiation is usually only

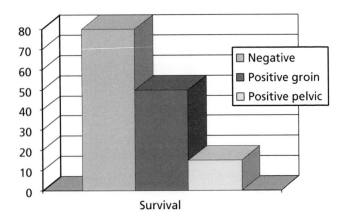

Figure 13.3 Survival in relation to nodal status

prescribed if two or more nodes are found to contain disease.[10,11] If there is complete macroscopic replacement or capsular breach then one node only will prompt postoperative radiotherapy. When nodes become grossly enlarged, fixed and/or ulcerated the decision may well be to treat first with radiotherapy, reserving surgical resection for those with an incomplete response. The management of grossly involved nodes is still a much-debated area of management with little in the way of controlled data to provide evidence on which care can be based. There may be a case, however, for using surgical resection first in situations where the nodes are still unfixed as this will theoretically debulk tumour and may enhance any subsequent response to radiotherapy.

If lymphadenectomy is deemed appropriate, the extent and laterality need to be judged on characteristics of the primary tumour thus the extent of the primary tumour becomes the next phase of assessment.

Staging of vulval cancer

The FIGO and TNM systems are used to describe the local, regional and distant extent of vulval cancer (see Appendix 1). Table 13.1 shows the equivalent stages in each system.

The approach to management differs for disease more extensive than stage II. In these advanced cases, there is a greater reliance on multidisciplinary treatment from the outset. In the early cases, surgery is the basis of treatment at the outset.[12,13] An example of this might be the use of radiotherapy or chemotherapy to reduce the volume (or occasionally eradicate disease) prior to surgery in an attempt to minimise morbidity and preserve function. The same approach might be used for

Table 13.1 FIGO and TNM staging for vulval cancer

FIGO stage	Description	TNM stage
I	Lesion < 2 cm confined to the vulva or perineum; no lymph node metastases	$T_1N_0M_0$
Ia	< 1 mm stromal invasion; lesion < 2 cm	
Ib	> 1 mm stromal invasion; lesion < 2 cm	
II	Tumour confined to the vulva or perineum, > 2 cm in maximal dimension	$T_2N_0M_0$
III	Tumour of any size arising on the vulva or perineum with: 1) adjacent spread to urethra, vagina or anus, or 2) unilateral groin node metastasis	$T_3N_0M_0$ $T_3N_1M_0$ $T_1N_1M_0$ $T_2N_1M_0$
IVa	Tumour invading any of the following: upper urethra, bladder mucosa, rectal mucosa; Pelvic bone and/or bilateral regional nodal metastases	$T_3N_2M_0$ $T_2N_2M_0$ $T_3N_2M_0$ T_4anyNM_0
IVb	Any distant metastasis, including pelvic lymph nodes	Any T Any N M_1

bulky nodes confirmed as positive although there are few data on which to base this type of management approach.

The stage of the tumour is not the only variable considered when constructing a management plan. Other variables include:

- tumour size and depth
- tumour location
- tumour histology
- co-morbidities
- patient's wishes.

CURRENT STANDARD
- All invasive squamous cancers other than stage Ia tumours will require some form of lymph node dissection.
- Lateralised T1 and T2 tumours may initially be managed by ipsilateral node dissection.
- Management of the primary tumour and the nodes should be decided on their own merits.

Managing the primary lesion

See also Chapter 5, Surgical principles.

Wide local excision has similar outcomes in terms of survival as does radical vulvectomy.[12,13] There is therefore no advantage in performing the more radical excision if the primary tumour can be widely excised. Wide excision should aim to achieve minimum clearance margins of 10 mm on all aspects of the tumour and should excise adjacent atypical skin, although probably not to the same depth. It becomes obvious that for a small, localised tumour, wide local excision is appropriate but, for large or multifocal lesions, complete removal of the vulva may still be required to meet these objectives.

CURRENT STANDARD
- Wide local excision is as effective as radical vulvectomy in early stage disease. All excision margins should be at least 10 mm.
- Preoperative radiation should be considered prior to excision if surgery is likely to compromise sphincter function.
- In large or multifocal lesions, radical vulvectomy may still be required to insure adequate excision margins.

If excision of the primary will result in compromise of the urethra, anus or, in some situations, removal of the clitoris, consideration should be given to prior treatment with radiation or chemoradiation. There are certainly some anecdotal data supporting this approach by demonstrating

Table 13.2   Treatment summary for vulval cancer

Disease extent	Description	Rx principle
Early disease	Stage I Lateral I and II Central, no sphincter compromise	WLE no nodes WLE, ipsilateral nodes WLE bilateral nodes, separate incisions
Advanced disease	Extensive vulval involvement	Primary radiotherapy to primary with groin node dissection
Metastatic	Clinically advanced disease	Excision ± chemoradiation Palliation may still require appropriate management of the primary

WLE = wide local excision

that less radical and often sphincter saving procedures can accomplish the desired excision after radiotherapy.[14-16] Table 13.2 shows a summary of treatment options for different stages of disease.

Management of the primary tumour and the nodes should be decided on their own merits.

Managing the lymph nodes

If the primary tumour is a basal cell carcinoma, a verrucous carcinoma, a superficially invasive squamous cell carcinoma[17] or a malignant melanoma with nonsuspicious nodes, then primary treatment does not include inguinofemoral lymphadenectomy. In all other cases it does. Available evidence suggests that in unifocal T1 and T2 tumours, an ipsilateral groin node dissection through a separate incision (i.e. not *en bloc*) should be performed.[18] The incidence of disease in the contralateral nodes is very low and only likely to be of clinical significance if there is already evidence of disease in the ipsilateral group. If this is the case, then a further procedure to remove the contralateral nodes will be required.

Local recurrence in the skin bridge (the tissue between the primary and groin nodes) is uncommon for T1 and T2 lesions.[19] Data on outcomes for larger lesions, or lesions with enlarged nodes, are not available. In these situations, *en bloc* resection of both groins is still regarded as the optimal approach to care.

If the primary lesion is a central tumour (wide excision would result in crossing the midline), then both groins should be resected. Again, separate incisions should be considered as optimal for T1 and possibly T2 lesions although no data support the separate incision approach when the primary is large and or there are clinically suspicious groin nodes.

TYPES OF GROIN NODE DISSECTION

The current consensus is that both the superficial inguinal and deep femoral nodes should be resected. Clinical research at present is identifying the so-called sentinel node. This is the node to which the tumour first drains. If this can be isolated (by radionuclide or dye injection) and resected, it can be assessed by frozen section pathology. If there is no evidence of tumour in this node, it would appear that the risk of metastases in the remainder of the chain is very low or zero, thus removing the need for any further dissection. The preliminary reports of this technique have been promising and larger trials are now in progress.[20]

PELVIC NODES

There is an increased risk of pelvic node disease in those proven to have disease in the groin nodes. Previously, this had been a prompt to extend the dissection to include those nodes around the iliac vessels. One randomised controlled trial, however, has suggested that patients who have their groin and pelvic nodes irradiated after a positive groin dissection fared better in terms of survival compared with those who had the groin and pelvic nodes resected.[10] The survival differences, however, can be ascribed to better control of relapse in the groin in the former group and not to improved control in the pelvis.

The case for resecting pelvic nodes is weak. One exception may be those cases where there is bulky disease at this site. Radiotherapy has been shown not to be particularly effective in controlling bulky disease in lymph nodes.

CURRENT STANDARD
- Inguinofemoral lymphadenectomy, either *en bloc* for large lesions or through separate groin incisions for early lesions, is the standard procedure.
- The pelvic nodes should be irradiated if the groin nodes require adjuvant radiotherapy.

Management of the primary tumour and the nodes should be decided on their own merits.

Early disease: adjuvant radiotherapy

Although it is the intention to treat with only surgery, there are situations where the risk of local relapse is felt to justify further or adjuvant treatment. This risk is only usually apparent after the examination of the excised primary and nodes.

INADEQUATE EXCISION MARGINS

If, on histological assessment, any excision margin is less than 8 mm, local radiation to the residual vulva or re-excision should be considered. The decision is usually based upon which of the two approaches is least likely to affect subsequent function. The smaller margin than that recommended for macroscopic excision takes into account shrinkage of the tissues following fixation.[12,13]

POSITIVE LYMPH NODES

Current convention is based upon observational series only. This dictates that adjuvant radiation should be prescribed to the groins and pelvic node groups if:

- more than one node shows microscopic disease
- one node is completely replaced by tumour
- one node demonstrates capsular breach.

ADJUVANT RADIATION

The prescribed dose is usually 45–50 Gy given to a depth of at least 8 cm. It is current practice to extend the fields to include the pelvic groups. Both sides should be considered for irradiation unless there is histological confirmation of negativity on one side.

CURRENT STANDARD
- More than one microscopically involved node, complete nodal replacement or capsular breach is an indication for adjuvant groin and pelvic node irradiation.
- Primary excision margins of less than 8 mm after fixation should prompt consideration of adjuvant local irradiation to the excision site or further excision.

Advanced vulval cancer

Advanced disease includes all patients with a vulval tumour where primary excision would compromise sphincter function. It also includes all patients where there is evidence of node involvement or distant metastasis.

Clinical assessment of nodal involvement is notoriously inaccurate and unless enlarged nodes are obviously malignant (Figures 13.4; plate 12: Figure 13.5; plate 13) (ulcerating or fungating) histological confirmation should always be sought. This can be achieved without recourse to major resection using fine-needle aspiration. If histological confirmation cannot be achieved then the primary approach should be by surgery.

MANAGEMENT OF GROSSLY INVOLVED NODES

There is no robust evidence to support either a primary surgical or primary radiotherapeutic approach. If surgery is used as the primary treatment modality, most, if not all, will require adjuvant radiotherapy. If radiotherapy is used as the primary approach it remains uncertain whether any further benefit accrues from a subsequent resection. Hypothetically, there would appear to be some logic in employing surgical debulking initially, if this were possible, and giving radiotherapy subsequently. Radiation is likely to be more effective if bulky, necrotic and hypoxic tissues are removed at the surgical procedure. Furthermore, this sequence of therapies would appear to be less likely to result in wound breakdown, as surgery would be performed on non-irradiated tissues.

COMBINED TREATMENT FOR THE PRIMARY

There have been several published series, albeit small, that would appear to support an approach of neoadjuvant radiotherapy in cases where the initial surgery would compromise function.[14-16] These series are summarised in Table 13.3. They all appear to demonstrate that vulval cancer is sensitive to radiation, that tumour shrinkage does occur and that, in some at least, less compromising surgery can then be performed. In both the Hacker et al.[14] and Rotmensch et al.[15] series, patients were included if, at the outset, a colostomy would have been required to accomplish complete tumour clearance. Hacker avoided a colostomy in all seven of his patients with an overall survival of 62% and Rotmench avoided colostomy in 6 of 16, with an overall survival of 45%. Whether these figures can be further improved with chemoradiation remains to be seen, although the toxicity of vulval irradiation is not inconsequential and likely to be greater with the addition of chemotherapy.

Some women will achieve a complete response following radiotherapy. Whether surgery is necessary or not in such cases is also largely speculative. Current practice is to perform multiple biopsies from the previously recorded tumour site three months following completion of therapy, only performing radical excision if there is histological evidence of residual disease. For partial responses, radical excision with the nodes is still standard practice.

Table 13.3   Published series supporting neoadjuvant radiotherapy in cases of vulval cancer where initial surgery would compromise function

Study	Cases (n)	Surgery	Residual tumour (%)	Survival (%)	Localised tumour (%)	Colostomy
Acosta et al.[21]	14	RV+N	70	62	nk	2
Hacker et al.[14]	7	RLE+(N)	40	62	14	0
Boronow et al.[16]	37	RLE+(N)	57	76	14	4
Carson et al.[22]	8	RLE**	25	25	nk	0
Rotmensch et al.[15]	16	RV+N	85	45	25	6
Wahlen et al.[23]	19	RLE	47	89	37	2
Lupi et al.[24]	24	RV+N	67	55	21	0

N = and inguinofemoral nodes; RLE = Radical local excision; RV = radical vulvectomy

Reconstructive surgery

Reconstructive surgery may be required because of large deficits that cannot be closed at the time of excision or because of a desire to retain as much function as possible and for cosmetic reasons. The requirement for reconstruction should be considered in all patients undergoing surgery for vulval cancer.

A variety of rotational and transposition grafts have been used in vulval reconstruction and this depends upon the site of the defect, its size and the availability of suitable graft sites. Split skin is also of value, particularly in areas where the bulk of a transposition graft might not be easily accommodated or where there is a high risk of graft breakdown such as in an infected site or in heavy smokers.

The increasing use of reconstruction in vulval cancer management has made reconstructive surgeons an integral part of the multidisciplinary team. Gynaecological oncologists should, however, be trained in basic techniques, which will suffice for the majority of patients.

CURRENT STANDARD
- In locally advanced tumours, preoperative radiation or chemoradiation should be considered in an attempt to reduce subsequent surgical morbidity.
- Reconstruction should be considered and discussed in all cases where radical excision is contemplated.

Morbidity

Morbidity results as a consequence of:

- relapsed disease (local, regional and distant)
- structural damage as a consequence of treatment
- psychosexual damage.

Either re-excision or radiation can manage local relapse and, generally, the modality that will result in least functional impairment should be the first choice. In women who have already been irradiated, the choice is usually limited to surgery. It is far preferable to try and avoid local recurrence by ensuring adequate excision margins at the outset. Reconstruction at the time of surgery is preferable if this allows wider margins and while preservation of function is important, this should not compromise cure.

Relapse in the groin is almost invariably incurable. Radiotherapy may be given if this has not been done so before and attempted excisions have also been tried. These patients invariably do badly and will die of their disease, which underlines the importance of appropriate management planning at the outset.

POSTOPERATIVE MORBIDITY

The high morbidity and long hospital stay traditionally associated with radical vulvectomy have largely driven the changes in care. While the more conservative approaches to management currently employed have improved morbidity, it is still seen more frequently than one would wish. The major postoperative morbidities are:

- wound breakdown
- wound infection
- deep-vein thrombosis and pulmonary embolism
- pressure sores.

Other morbidity becomes apparent at follow-up and this is one reason why follow-up is still considered important in this disease. The problems that may arise include:

- introital stenosis
- incontinence (urinary and faecal)
- rectocele
- lymphocyst
- lymphoedema
- hernia
- psychosexual problems.

SUMMARY
- Vulval cancer is uncommon and requires a truly multidisciplinary approach in order to offer high quality and effective care.
- Vulval cancer should only be managed in cancer centres that offer the full range of expertise that patients suffering from the disease require.
- The principles of care are directed at maximising disease control and minimising morbidity.
- The fact that patients are usually elderly and often have significant co-morbidity should not provide obstacles or indeed excuses for inadequate disease planning.
- Developments in the future are likely to address the problems of both diagnosis and treatment of disease in the regional node groups thus further reducing morbidity.

References

1. Penney GC, Kitchener HC, Templeton A. *The management of carcinoma of the vulva: current opinion and current practice among consultant gynaecologists in Scotland.* Health Bulletin 1995; 53(1).

2. Rhodes CA, Cummins C, Shafi M. The management of squamous cell vulval cancer: a population based retrospective study of 411 cases. *Br J Obstet Gynaecol* 1998; **105**: 200–5.

3. Van der Velden J, van Lindert ACM, Gimbrere CHF, Oosting H, Heintz APM. Epidemiologic data on vulvar cancer: comparison of hospital with population based data. *Gynecol Oncol* 1996; **62**: 379–83.

4. Jones RW, Baranyai J, Stables S. Trends in squamous cell carcinoma of the vulva: the influence of vulvar intraepithelial neoplasia. *Obstet Gynecol* 1997; **90**: 448–52.

5. Herod JJO, Shafi MI, Rollason TP, Jordan JA, Luesley DM. Vulvar intraepithelial neoplasia: long term follow up of treated ,untreated women. *Br J Obstet Gynaecol* 1996; **103**: 446–52.

6. Fishman DA, Chambers SK, Shwartz PE, Kohorn EL, Chambers JT. Extramammary Paget's disease of the vulva. *Gynecol Oncol* 1995; **56**: 266–70.

7. Ragnarssonolding B, Johanson H, Rutgvist LE, Ringborg U. Malignant melanoma of the vulva, vagina: trends in incidence, age distribution, long term survival among 245 consecutive cases in Sweden 1960–1984. *Cancer* 1993; **71**: 1893–7.

8. Bradgate M, Rollason TP, McConkey CC, Powe UJ. Malignant melanoma of the vulva: A clinico-pathological study of 50 cases. *Br J Obstet Gynaecol* 1990; **97**: 124–33.

9. Friedrich EG. Vulvar dystrophy. *Clin Obstet Gynecol* 1985; **28**: 178–87.

10. Homesley H, Bundy BN, Sedlis A, Adcock L. Radiation therapy versus pelvic node resection for carcinoma of the vulva with positive groin nodes. *Obstet Gynecol* 1986; **68**: 733–40.

11. Van der Velden J, van Lindert ACM, Lammes FB, ten Kate FJW, Sie-Go DMDS, Oosting H, *et al.* Extracapsular growth of lymph node metastases in squamous cell carcinoma of the vulva. *Cancer* 1995; **75**: 2885–90.

12. Heaps JM, Yao SF, Montz FJ, Hacker NF, Bereck JS. Surgical-pathological variables predictive of local recurrence in squamous cell carcinoma of the vulva. *Gynecol Oncol* 1990; **38**: 309–14.

13. Hacker NF, Van der Velden J. Conservative management of early vulvar cancer. *Cancer* 1993; **71**: 1673–7.

14. Hacker NF, Berek JS, Juillard JF, Lagasse LD. Pre-operative radiotherapy for locally advanced vulvar cancer. *Cancer* 1984; **54**: 2056–61.

15. Rotmensch J, Rubin SJ, Sutton HG, Javaheri G, Halpern HJ, Schwartz JL, *et al.* Preoperative radiotherapy followed by radical vulvectomy with inguinal lymphadenectomy for advanced vulvar carcinomas. *Gynecol Oncol* 1990; **36**: 181–4.

16. Boronow RC, Hickman BT, Reagan MT, Smith A, Steadman RE. Combined therapy as an alternative to exenteration for locally advanced vulvovaginal cancer. *Am J Clin Oncol* 1987; **10**: 171–81.

17. Sedlis A, Homesley H, Bundy BN, Marshall R, Yordan E, Hacker N, *et al.* Positive groin lymph nodes in superficial squamous cell vulvar cancer. *Am J Obstet Gynecol* 1987; **156**: 1159–64.

18. Stehman FB, Bundy BN, Dvoretsky PM, Creasman WT. Early stage I carcinoma of the vulva treated with ipsilateral superficial inguinal lymphadenectomy and modified radical hemivulvectomy. A prospective study of the Gynecologic Oncology Group. *Obstet Gynecol* 1992; **79**: 490–7.

19. Hacker NF, Leuchter RS, Bereck JS, Castaldo TW, Lagasse LD. Radical vulvectomy and bilateral inguinal lymphadenectomy through separate groin incisions. *Obstet Gynecol* 1981; **58**: 574–9.

20. Decesare SL, Fiorica JV, Roberts WS, Reintgen D, Arango H, Hoffman MS, *et al.* A pilot study utilising intraoperative lymphoscintigraphy for identification of the sentinel lymph nodes in vulvar cancer. *Gynecol Oncol* 1997; **66**: 425–8.

21. Acosta AA, Given FT, Frazier AB, Cordoba RB, Luninari A. Preoperative radiation therapy in the management of squamous cell carcinoma of the vulva: a preliminary report. *Am J Obstet Gynecol* 1978; **132**: 198–206.

22. Carson LF, Twiggs LB, Adcock LL, Prem KA, Potish RA. Multimodality therapy for advanced and recurrent vulvar squamous cell carcinoma: a pilot project. *J Reprod Med* 1990; **35**: 1029–32.

23. Wahlen SA, Slater JD, Wagner RJ, Wang WA, Keeney ED, Hocko JM, *et al.* Concurrent radiation therapy and chemotherapy in the treatment of primary squamous cell carcinoma of the vulva. *Cancer* 1995; **75**: 2289–94.

24. Lupi G, Raspagliesi F, Zucali R, Fontanelli R, Paladini D, Kenda R, *et al.* Combined pre-operative chemoradiotherapy followed by radical surgery in locally advanced vulvar carcinoma. *Cancer* 1996; **77**: 1472–8.

14 Uncommon gynaecological cancers

Introduction

The investigation and management of uncommon gynaecological cancers is based mainly upon cohort studies, case series and expert opinion. The evidence base is weak, with few randomised controlled trials available to guide the treatment of these tumours, due to their rarity. However, the management of gestational trophoblastic disease is more robust as randomised controlled trials have been undertaken and treatment modified accordingly.

Gestational trophoblastic disease

Gestational trophoblastic disease (GTD) is defined as an excessive and inappropriate proliferation of the trophoblast. It includes a spectrum of disease from the benign hydatidiform mole (complete and partial), to the malignant gestational trophoblastic tumour (GTT), i.e. invasive mole, choriocarcinoma and the rare placental site trophoblastic tumour (PSTT).

Complete moles occur in about one per 1000 pregnancies and partial hydatidiform moles in three per 1000 pregnancies. Complete moles lack identifiable embryonic or fetal tissue and usually have a diploid 46XX karyotype, with entirely paternal chromosomes. Partial hydatidiform moles have identifiable embryonic or fetal tissue and usually have a triploid karyotype (69 chromosomes), with an extra haploid set of paternal chromosomes.

The risk of developing malignant disease after suction evacuation of a complete mole is 15% (with metastases in 4%) and 2–4% of patients after evacuation of a partial hydatidiform mole. The malignant tumour is usually an invasive mole, but choriocarcinoma can arise in up to 3% of complete moles and, rarely, after a partial hydatidiform mole.

Invasive moles invade the myometrium and are characterised by trophoblastic hyperplasia and the persistence of placental villous structures. In virtually all cases they are preceded by a molar pregnancy and rarely progress to choriocarcinoma. They can metastasise to the lungs, vagina, brain, liver and, rarely, the skin, lymph nodes and bone. It does not progress like a true cancer and often regresses spontaneously.

Choriocarcinoma arises from the trophoblast and contains both cytotrophoblast and syncytiotrophoblast. The lack of villous structures distinguishes it from an invasive mole. Choriocarcinoma can arise from any pregnancy, which may have occurred up to several years previously. More than 50% are preceded by a molar pregnancy and they are 1000 times more common after a complete mole than a normal pregnancy. They can metastasise.

Placental site trophoblastic tumour arises from the trophoblast of the placental bed and consists of mainly cytotrophoblastic cells, hence the relatively low level of hCG associated with this tumour. Human placental lactogen can be detected in both serum and immunohistochemically on histology. It is a rare, with one case of PSTT for every 100 cases of invasive mole and choriocarcinoma. Treatment is by complete surgical excision as it is not a chemosensitive tumour.

Table 14.1 Signs and symptoms of complete molar pregnancy

Symptom	Occurrence (%)	Description
Vaginal bleeding		May cause anaemia; vesicles may also be passed vaginally
Excessive uterine size	≤ 50	Usually associated with very high levels of hCG, which may be > 200 000
Hyperemesis gravidarum		Due to the increased levels of hCG; may result in severe electrolyte disturbances
Toxaemia		Pre-eclampsia is also associated with an increased level of hCG; complete mole should be considered in any woman developing hypertension in the first trimester
Hyperthyroidism	c. 7	thought to be due to the thyrotropic activity of hCG
Trophoblastic embolisation	≤ 2%	Patients may have chest pain, tachypnoea, tachycardia and respiratory distress requiring cardiopulmonary support
Theca lutein ovarian cysts	≤ 50 (> 6 cm diameter)	Usually bilateral and multilocular and associated with markedly elevated serum hCG levels; normally regress spontaneously within 2–4 months, after evacuation

FIGO STAGING OF GESTATIONAL TROPHOBLASTIC TUMOURS

In 1991, FIGO added nonsurgical pathologic prognostic risk factors to the anatomical staging system (see Appendix 1). Risk factors affecting staging include urinary hCG levels > 100 000 miu/ml and/or serum βhCG > 40000 miu/ml and the duration of disease more than six months from termination of the antecedent pregnancy.

RISK FACTORS

Risk factors for GTD include:

- maternal age: teenagers have a slightly higher incidence than women aged 20–40 years and women over 40 years of age have a much higher incidence
- race: Asians have higher rates of GTD than Arabs and Caucasians, with African Americans having a low incidence
- reproductive history: women who have had a previous molar pregnancy are at much greater risk of another compared with women who have never had a molar pregnancy
- parental blood groups: women with blood group A and whose partners are blood group O have a higher risk of choriocarcinoma
- genetic predisposition: familial clustering of GTD has been reported.

There are no environmental factors associated with GTD.

PRESENTATION AND DIAGNOSIS

Patients with a partial hydatidiform mole usually present with the signs and symptoms of an incomplete or missed miscarriage. The diagnosis is often made on histology of the retained products of conception.

Complete molar pregnancies present with signs and symptoms shown in Table 14.1. The diagnosis of a complete mole is now often made in the first trimester, either by the detection of raised hCG levels or by the classic vesicular 'snowstorm' ultrasound appearance.

INVESTIGATIONS

Preoperative investigations include:

- history and examination
- pelvic ultrasound scan
- FBC/clotting – to exclude anaemia or clotting disorder
- U&Es/liver function tests/thyroid function tests – to exclude metastatic disease or hyperthyroidism
- crossmatch blood – as there is a risk of haemorrhage at evacuation.

MANAGEMENT

Suction evacuation of the uterine cavity is the treatment of choice for molar pregnancy. This should be performed by an experienced surgeon, as there is an increased risk of perforation and haemorrhage. All tissue should be sent for histological examination.

After evacuation patients should be registered with a UK supraregional centre (Charing Cross Hospital, London; Weston Park Hospital, Sheffield; or Ninewells Hospital, Dundee) and computerised hCG follow-up undertaken. Weekly serial hCG measurements should be taken until the level has returned to normal for four weeks. If the level reaches normal within eight weeks of the diagnosis of molar pregnancy, follow-up is undertaken for six months, otherwise it is continued for two years. Patients should use effective contraception for six months following an evacuation for a molar pregnancy, to avoid confusion between a normal pregnancy and a rising hCG titre, indicating the development of invasive disease. Oral contraceptives can be used as they do not increases the risk of post-molar trophoblastic disease.[1] hCG levels should be taken at six and 12 weeks post-delivery after any future pregnancy due to the increased risk of trophoblastic disease.

Approximately 8% of women registered in the UK with GTD will need adjuvant chemotherapy. The use of prophylactic chemotherapy in patients who are unlikely to comply with follow-up is controversial. There is a theoretical risk that such patients will develop drug resistance should they require chemotherapy for GTT in the future.

The World Health Organization Scientific Group agreed in 1983 that chemotherapy should be given to patients who have had a partial hydatidiform mole when:

- a high level of hCG is present four weeks after evacuation: serum level > 20000 iu/l, urine level > 30000 iu/l (due to the risk of uterine perforation)
- rising hCG levels at any time post-evacuation
- histological identification of choriocarcinoma or evidence of central nervous system, renal, hepatic or gastrointestinal metastases, or pulmonary metastases > 2 cm in diameter or greater than three in number.

Charing Cross Hospital, London, will also give chemotherapy to patients with persistent uterine haemorrhage or detectable hCG in serum or urine four to six months post-evacuation.

A number of prognostic variables have been identified and patients can be categorised into low-, medium- and high-risk,[2] so that their treatment is stratified appropriately. This ranges from single agent methotrexate plus folinic acid, etoposide or actinomycin D to intensive drug combinations, e.g. EMA-CO (actinomycin D, etoposide, methotrexate, folinic acid, vincristine and cyclophosphamide). Charing Cross Hospital uses a modification of Bagshawe's prognostic scoring system.

Hysterectomy with adjuvant single-agent chemotherapy may be appropriate treatment for stage I GTD in patients who do not wish to preserve fertility. It may also be required to control uterine haemorrhage or sepsis with metastatic GTT. In patients with drug resistant disease, where the active site can be identified, salvage surgery is indicated. Success rates for salvage surgery are hysterectomy (15%), thoracotomy (43%) and craniotomy (71%).

FOLLOW-UP AND OUTCOME POST-CHEMOTHERAPY

After completion of chemotherapy, patients are followed-up by serial serum and urine hCG estimations. Patients are advised against pregnancy for a year after completing chemotherapy, to distinguish between a further pregnancy and relapsed disease. Patients with a complete molar pregnancy can anticipate normal future reproductive function, with up to 77.5% having live births following chemotherapy. However, patients who have had one molar pregnancy have a 1% risk of a further molar pregnancy.[3] Chemotherapy with etoposide may increase the rate of second tumours, such as acute myeloid leukaemia.

The long-term survival of patients treated for gestational trophoblastic tumour at Charing Cross Hospital is 94% at 15-year follow-up.

Cancer of the fallopian tube

Primary carcinoma of the fallopian tube is rare, accounting for 0.3% of all gynaecological malignancies. The majority of cancers are epithelial in origin, commonly serous but, rarely, sarcomas occur. Most tubal malignancies are secondary from the uterus, ovary, gastrointestinal tract or breast.

Tubal cancers occur most frequently in the fifth and sixth decades, with a mean age of 55–60 years. Many patients are nulliparous (45%) and many have a history of infertility.

FIGO STAGING OF CARCINOMA OF THE FALLOPIAN TUBE

Staging for fallopian tube carcinoma is by the surgical pathological system (see Appendix 1). Operative findings prior to tumour debulking may be modified by histopathological, clinical or radiological evaluation.

PRESENTATION AND DIAGNOSIS

Primary adenocarcinoma of the fallopian tube can present with variable, non-specific symptoms:

- abdominal pain
- serosanguinous discharge (hydrops tubae profluens)
- pelvic mass

This triad of symptoms occurs in < 15% of patients.

- abnormal vaginal bleeding, often postmenopausal
- unexplained abnormal cervical cytology
- urinary or bowel disturbance.

Fallopian tube cancer is bilateral in 10–20% of cases and is often found incidentally in asymptomatic women at the time of total abdominal hysterectomy and bilateral salpingo-oophorectomy (Figures 14.1; plate 13: Figure 14.2; plate 14). Many present with early disease: 37% with stage I and 20% with stage II disease, respectively. Therefore, the overall five-year survival rate for fallopian tube carcinoma is higher than that for epithelial ovarian cancer, which presents much later.

INVESTIGATIONS

- Serum CA125 levels: these may be elevated in tubal carcinoma; CA125 titres may predict tumour presence and can monitor response to therapy.
- Routine preoperative tests required for any laparotomy for suspected gynaecological malignancy (full blood count, U&Es, liver function tests, chest X-ray).
- Pelvic/abdominal ultrasound scan.
- CT scan pelvis/abdomen may be useful to delineate tumour.

MANAGEMENT

Laparotomy
The treatment of fallopian tube carcinoma is identical to that of epithelial ovarian carcinoma (see Chapter 5). Primary debulking surgery is performed to stage the disease and to attempt total macroscopic clearance. Unilateral salpingo-oophorectomy may be performed in young women with a stage IA well-differentiated tumour who are desirous of fertility.

Chemotherapy
Adjuvant cisplatin-based combination chemotherapy has been used in tubal carcinoma with up to an 80% response rate. Due to the clinical and histological similarity between tubal and epithelial ovarian cancer patients, response rates and survival to chemotherapy are expected to be

similar in the two groups. Currently, combination carboplatin and paclitaxel would be recommended (see also Chapter 8).

Radiation
Radiation therapy has frequently been used in the treatment of fallopian tube carcinoma in the past. However, the role of radiation in the management of this disease remains unclear. Whole-abdomen irradiation may improve survival in patients with completely resected disease or microscopic metastases[4] (see also Chapter 7).

TUBAL SARCOMAS

Tubal sarcomas, mainly malignant mixed mesodermal tumours, are very rare. They usually present at an advanced stage in the sixth decade. Treatment is by primary debulking surgery and adjuvant combination chemotherapy. The overall five-year survival rate for patients with epithelial tubal carcinomas is 56%. The five-year survival rates for patients, according to stage at presentation, are 84% for stage I, 52% for stage II and 36% for stage III disease, respectively.

Nonepithelial ovarian cancers

Nonepithelial malignancies of the ovary account for approximately 10% of all ovarian cancers. They include germ cell malignancies, sex cord-stromal tumours, metastatic carcinomas to the ovary and the rare lipoid cell tumours, sarcomas and small-cell carcinomas of the ovary.

OVARIAN GERM CELL TUMOURS

Germ cell tumours are derived from the primordial germ cells of the ovary. Although 20–30% of all ovarian neoplasms (both benign and malignant) are of germ cell origin, only approximately 3% are malignant. However, in the first two decades of life, almost 70% of ovarian tumours are of germ cell origin, and one-third of these are malignant. Ovarian germ cell tumours are staged as for epithelial ovarian carcinoma and are classified according to histological type (Table 14.2).

Some ovarian germ cell malignancies secrete hormones detectable in the serum.

- Dysgerminomas secrete placental alkaline phosphatase and lactate dehydrogenase.
- Endodermal sinus tumour secretes alphafetoprotein (AFP).
- Embryonal carcinoma secretes AFP and hCG.
- Choriocarcinoma secretes hCG.

Table 14.2 Histological typing of ovarian germ cell tumours

Class	Type
1	Dysgerminoma

2	Teratoma:
	    A. Immature
	    B. Mature: (1) Solid
	                 (2) Cystic a. Dermoid cyst (mature cystic teratoma)
	                                b. Dermoid cyst with malignant transformation
	    C. Monodermal and highly specialised:
	                 (1) Struma ovarii
	                 (2) Carcinoid
	                 (3) Struma ovarii and carcinoid
	                 (4) Others

3	Endodermal sinus tumour
4	Embryonal carcinoma
5	Polyembryona
6	Choriocarcinoma
7	Mixed forms

Presentation and diagnosis

Germ cell malignancies grow rapidly and often present with pelvic pain due to capsular distension, haemorrhage or necrosis. The rapidly enlarging pelvic mass may cause bowel or bladder pressure symptoms or menstrual irregularities. Diagnosis can be delayed by a misdiagnosis of pregnancy.

A germ cell tumour should be suspected prior to surgery in a young woman with a predominately solid ovarian tumour; such patients should be referred to a gynaecological oncologist.

Investigations

- Full blood count
- U&Es
- Liver function tests
- Chest X-ray
- Pelvic/abdominal ultrasound scan
- CT scan pelvis/abdomen to exclude retroperitoneal lymphadenopathy and liver metastases
- hCG
- AFP
- Karyotype: premenarchal ovarian germ cell tumours often arise in dysgenetic gonads.

DYSGERMINOMAS

Dysgerminomas account for approximately 30–40% of all ovarian germ cell tumours, representing only 1–3% of all ovarian cancers. However, they do account for 5–10% of ovarian cancers in patients under 20 years of age, with 75% of dysgerminomas occurring between 10 and 30 years of age.[5] Approximately 5% are found in patients with a female phenotype and abnormal glands. Bilateral tumours are found in 10–15% and 75% of patients are stage I at presentation.

Management

Stage IA disease can be treated conservatively with unilateral salpingo-oophorectomy, providing appropriate staging has been undertaken to exclude occult metastatic disease. Advanced disease is treated by total abdominal hysterectomy and bilateral salpingo-oophorectomy and all patients with a Y chromosome on karyotyping should have a bilateral oophorectomy.

Dysgerminomas are radiation-sensitive but chemotherapy has replaced radiotherapy to preserve fertility (see also Chapter 8). Advanced-stage or incompletely resected dysgerminomas are treated with four cycles of BEP. In patients with recurrent disease who have received prior BEP chemotherapy, POMB-ACE (cisplatin, vincristine, methotrexate, and bleomycin; and actinomycin D, cyclophosphamide and etoposide) may be used.

Outcome

Patients with stage IA dysgerminomas treated by unilateral salpingo-oophorectomy have a five-year survival rate greater than 95%. Combination chemotherapy now achieves cure rates of 90–100% for advanced disease.[6]

IMMATURE TERATOMAS

Immature teratomas contain elements that resemble tissues derived from the embryo. Pure immature teratomas account for 10–20% of all ovarian malignancies in patients aged less than 20 years of age. Malignant transformation of a mature teratoma occurs in 0.5–2.0% of tumours, commonly to squamous cell carcinoma but, rarely, to adenocarcinomas, primary melanomas or carcinoid tumours. Immature teratomas are classified according to a grading system (grades 1 to 3), based upon the degree of differentiation and the quantity of immature tissue. Tumours with malignant squamous elements have a poorer prognosis.

Premenopausal patients with disease confined to a single ovary are treated by unilateral salpingo-oophorectomy with surgical staging. Contralateral ovarian involvement is rare. Patients with stage IA, grade 1 tumours do not require adjuvant therapy. All other stages are treated with adjuvant BEP combination chemotherapy (see also Chapter 8). Radiation is reserved for patients with localized persistent disease post-chemotherapy (see Chapter 7).

The most important prognostic feature of immature teratomas is the grade of the lesion.[7] The overall five-year survival rate for pure immature teratomas is 70–80%.

ENDODERMAL SINUS TUMOUR

Endodermal sinus tumours are derived from the primitive yolk sac. The median age at presentation is 18 years and approximately one-third of cases are premenarchal. Abdominal and/or pelvic pain occurs in 75% and 10% have an asymptomatic pelvic mass. Most endodermal sinus tumours secrete AFP, rarely, they secrete α_1-antitrypsin.

The surgical treatment of endodermal sinus tumour is unilateral salpingo-oophorectomy, with frozen section for diagnosis. The addition of hysterectomy and contralateral salpingo-oophorectomy does not alter outcome.[5] Surgical staging is not indicated as all patients require either adjuvant or therapeutic combination chemotherapy with BEP or POMB-ACE. Survival has improved significantly with the introduction of routine combination chemotherapy, with two-year survival now greater than 70%.

EMBRYONAL CARCINOMA

Embryonal carcinoma of the ovary is extremely rare and is distinguished from choriocarcinoma of the ovary by the absence of syncytiotrophoblastic and cytotrophoblastic cells. The median age at presentation is 14 years and patients may present with signs of precocious pseudopuberty as the tumours may secrete oestrogens. These tumours frequently secrete AFP and hCG. Management is as for endodermal sinus tumours, i.e. unilateral salpingo-oophorectomy and adjuvant BEP chemotherapy.

POLYEMBRYOMA

Polyembryoma of the ovaries is extremely rare, occurring in very young premenarchal girls. The tumour is composed of 'embryoid bodies', consisting of endoderm, mesoderm and ectoderm and secretes AFP and hCG. Chemotherapy with VAC (vincristine, actinomycin D and cyclophosphamide) has been reported to be effective.

CHORIOCARCINOMA OF THE OVARY

Pure non-gestational choriocarcinoma of the ovary is also extremely rare. Most patients are aged less than 20 years and have metastases at presentation. Treatment is with chemotherapy but the prognosis is poor.

MIXED GERM CELL TUMOURS

Mixed germ cell tumours of the ovary contain two or more elements of the previously described germ cell tumours. The most frequent combination is dysgerminoma and endodermal sinus tumour. The tumours may secrete AFP or hCG, depending on the components. Treatment is with combination BEP chemotherapy. The most important prognostic features are the size of the primary tumour and the relative amount of the most malignant component. Stage IA lesions of less than 10 cm have a 100% survival rate.

OVARIAN SEX CORD–STROMAL CELL TUMOURS

Sex cord–stromal tumours account for 5–8% of all ovarian malignancies.[5] These tumours are derived from the sex cords and the ovarian stroma or mesenchyme, and include the 'female' cells (i.e. granulose and theca cells) and 'male' cells (i.e. Sertoli and Leydig cells).

GRANULOSA–STROMAL CELL TUMOURS

Granulosa–stromal cell tumours include granulose cell tumours, thecomas and fibromas. The granulosa cell tumour is a low-grade malignancy. Thecomas and fibromas are rarely malignant and are then referred to as fibrosarcomas.

GRANULOSA CELL TUMOURS

Granulosa cell tumours secrete oestrogen and occur in women of all ages. Five percent are found in prepubertal girls and are associated with sexual pseudoprecocity. In women of reproductive age they present with menstrual irregularity, secondary amenorrhoea or endometrial cystic hyperplasia. Postmenopausal bleeding is a common feature due to oestrogenic stimulation of the endometrium. Endometrial cancer occurs in at least 5% of cases of granulose cell tumour and 25–50% are associated with endometrial hyperplasia. Rarely, they may produce androgens and cause virilisation. They are bilateral in 2% of cases.

Granulosa cell tumours may present like any ovarian tumour but tend to be haemorrhagic, occasionally rupturing and causing a haemoperitoneum. They usually present as stage I disease but may recur 5–30 years after initial diagnosis, with lung, liver or brain metastases.

Inhibin is secreted by granulose cell tumours and is a useful marker for the disease.

Management

The treatment of granulosa cell tumours depends upon the age of the patient and the extent of the disease. Stage IA tumours in patients desirous of fertility are treated by unilateral salpingo-oophorectomy. In women not wanting fertility, a total abdominal hysterectomy and bilateral salpingo-oophorectomy is performed. If the uterus is left *in situ*, a dilatation and curettage of the uterus should be performed to exclude a coexistent adenocarcinoma of the endometrium.

Adjuvant chemotherapy with BEP is used to treat recurrent or metastatic disease. Pelvic radiation may help to palliate isolated pelvic recurrences.[8] The ten-year survival rate for granulosa cell tumours is greater than 90%; at 20 years, the survival rate falls to 75%.

SERTOLI–LEYDIG TUMOURS

Sertoli–Leydig tumours consist of Sertoli cells, Leydig cells and fibroblasts in varying proportions. They account for 0.5% of all ovarian cancers and are usually low-grade malignancies. Seventy-five percent occur in women less than 40 years of age and they often cause virilisation due to androgen secretion (oligomenorrhoea, breast atrophy, acne, hirsutism, clitoromegaly, deepening of the voice and temporal baldness).

Management is with unilateral salpingo-oophorectomy and evaluation of the contralateral ovary is adequate treatment in patients desirous of fertility. Older patients are usually treated by total abdominal hysterectomy and bilateral salpingo-oophorectomy. Pelvic radiation and VAC chemotherapy have also been used in this disease. The five-year survival rate is 70–90%.

Transitional cell (Brenner) tumours of the ovary

Brenner tumours account for 1–2% of all ovarian tumours. They are bilateral in 10–15% of cases and commonly present in the fifth and sixth decades. They arise from wolffian metaplasia of the ovarian surface epithelium and consist of islands of transitional epithelium (Walthard nests) in dense fibrous stroma. Most tumours are less than 2 cm in diameter.

Brenner tumours are commonly benign but may be borderline and, rarely, malignant. Malignant Brenner tumours are defined by coexistence of a benign Brenner tumour component and a transitional cell carcinoma. These tumours can secrete oestrogen and often present with abnormal vaginal bleeding. The prognosis is good if the tumour is confined to the ovary.

Vaginal cancer

Primary carcinoma of the vagina accounts for 1–2% of gynaecological malignancies. Most vaginal carcinomas are secondary, usually from the cervix, endometrium, colon or rectum, and occasionally from the ovary or vulva. Squamous cell carcinoma is the most common type of vaginal cancer, with a mean age at presentation of 60 years. Approximately 9% of primary vaginal carcinomas are adenocarcinomas, which usually present in younger women. Vaginal sarcomas are extremely rare and are treated by surgical excision.

RISK FACTORS

- CIN or cervical carcinoma: up to 30% of primary vaginal cancers occur in patients with a history of preinvasive or invasive cervical cancer.[9]
- VAIN: this is known to be a precursor but its malignant potential is unknown.[10]
- Exposure to diethylstilbestrol *in utero*: the risk of clear cell adenocarcinoma of the vagina in exposed female offspring is one in 1000 between birth and age 34 years.[11] Approximately 70% of vaginal adenocarcinomas are stage I at diagnosis.

FIGO STAGING OF CARCINOMA OF THE VAGINA

Staging of vaginal carcinoma is clinical, involving examination under anaesthesia, with combined rectovaginal examination, full thickness biopsy, cystoscopy, sigmoidoscopy and radiological investigation (see Appendix 1).

PRESENTATION AND DIAGNOSIS

Most patients present with vaginal bleeding or discharge (Figure 14.3: plate 14). Other symptoms include dysuria, urinary frequency, pelvic pain or pelvic mass and tenesmus. Careful inspection of the vaginal walls while withdrawing the bivalve speculum is required to identify the tumour, which is commonly present in the upper one-third of the vagina and easily missed on examination.

INVESTIGATIONS

- Full blood count
- U&Es
- Liver function tests
- Chest X-ray
- Pelvic/abdominal ultrasound scan
- Intravenous urogram
- CT/MRI of abdomen and pelvis.

MANAGEMENT

There is no consensus as to the correct management of primary vaginal cancer. Treatment is individualised and for most patients maintenance of a functional vagina is important.

Radiotherapy

Most patients are treated with radiotherapy consisting of a combination of teletherapy (external beam radiotherapy) and brachytherapy (intracavity or interstitial therapy). The mid-tumour dose should be at least 75 Gy and complications occur in 10–20% of cases. Vaginal necrosis may occur and vaginal stenosis occurs in between 13–48%. If the lower one-third of the vagina is involved, the inguinal nodes should be treated or dissected.

Surgery

Surgery has a limited role in the management of patients with vaginal cancer. It is considered in:

- stage I disease involving the upper posterior vagina – involves radical hysterectomy, partial vaginectomy and bilateral pelvic lymphadenectomy
- small, low, mobile stage I tumours – involves vulvectomy with inguinal lymphadenectomy
- young patients who require radiotherapy – pretreatment laparotomy allows ovarian transposition, surgical staging and resection of enlarged lymph nodes
- stage IVa disease, particularly if rectovaginal or vesicovaginal fistula present – pelvic exenteration may be appropriate
- patients with a central recurrence after radiotherapy often require pelvic exenteration.

The complications of vaginectomy for vaginal cancer include:

- haemorrhage
- trauma to bladder or rectum
- fixity of bladder base – scarring of bladder base can fix the urethra causing retention or urinary incontinence
- loss of all or part of the vagina
- shortening and scarring of the vagina – may require skin grafting
- fistulae formation
- chemotherapy.

Combined chemoradiation has been used as first-line treatment for advanced disease and palliative chemotherapy for recurrent disease. Experience is limited and has included the use of 5-flurouracil, mitomycin-C and cisplatin.[12]

OUTCOME

The five-year survival rates for vaginal carcinoma is 64–90% for stage I disease, 29–66% for stage II disease and 17–49% for stage III disease. The wide ranges in the reported five-year survival rates are probably related to the small numbers of cases in the reported series.

Uterine sarcomas

Uterine sarcomas are mesodermal tumours and account for 3–5% of all uterine cancers. They are a heterogeneous group of tumours without standardized treatment protocols. Criteria for histopathological classification also vary but the number of mitoses per ten high-power fields appears to be the most reliable predictor of tumour behaviour. The three most common malignant uterine sarcomas are leiomyosarcomas, endometrial stromal sarcomas and mixed mesodermal sarcomas.

RISK FACTORS

- More common in black women
- Previous pelvic irradiation.

STAGING OF UTERINE SARCOMAS

No staging system for uterine sarcomas has been proposed by FIGO, but a clinical staging system based upon that for endometrial carcinoma is often used (Table 14.3).

PRESENTATION AND DIAGNOSIS

Leiomyosarcomas usually arise *de novo* from uterine smooth muscle but 5–10% develop in a pre-existing fibroid, which may present with rapid enlargement. Patients may also present with pain, abnormal uterine bleeding or a pelvic abdominal mass. Leiomyosarcomas can be diagnosed on endometrial curettage but more than 80% are diagnosed incidentally at hysterectomy.

Table 14.3 Staging of uterine sarcoma	
Stage	Description
I	Sarcoma confined to the uterus
II	Sarcoma involving the corpus and cervix
III	Sarcoma spreading beyond the uterus, but not outside the pelvis
IV	Sarcoma spreading outside the pelvis or into the bladder or rectum

Endometrial stromal sarcomas are derived from the stromal cells of the endometrium and account for 15–20% of uterine sarcomas. They are premenopausal in more than 50% of patients and they usually present with abnormal vaginal bleeding. Low-grade stromal sarcomas have fewer than five mitoses per ten high-power fields and although they grow slowly, late recurrence can occur. High-grade stromal sarcomas, with fewer than ten mitoses per ten high-power fields, are aggressive tumours with an overall survival of less than 50%. Most are diagnosed at endometrial curettage.

Mixed mesodermal tumours (Figure 14.4: plate 15) usually occur in post-menopausal women who present with vaginal bleeding and often the tumour is seen protruding through the cervical os like a polyp.

MANAGEMENT

Uterine sarcomas are treated by surgical excision. This typically involves total abdominal hysterectomy and bilateral salpingo-oophorectomy, but young women with a leiomyosarcoma may have ovarian preservation. Adjuvant radiotherapy is considered to improve tumour control in the pelvis and may improve survival in surgical stage I or II disease.[13] Complete response rates of up to 8% have been achieved with adjuvant chemotherapy with doxorubicin, cisplatin and ifosfamide.

OUTCOME

The five-year survival rate for malignant uterine sarcomas is approximately 50%. There is no difference in five-year survival rates for the three main histological types, when corrected for stage of disease at presentation.

Paediatric oncology

Gynaecological malignancy is uncommon in childhood and adolescence. If suspected, patients should be referred to a gynaecological oncologist due to the rarity of the tumour. Neonatal cancers are usually embryonic tumours, with sarcomas presenting in adolescence.

OVARIAN TUMOURS

Ovarian tumours are the most common gynaecological tumours in girls but account for no more than 1% of all tumours in girls under 16 years of age. About 30% of childhood ovarian tumours are benign teratomas. The most common malignant ovarian tumours in childhood are germ-cell carcinomas, i.e., dysgerminoma, endodermal sinus tumour, malignant teratoma and, more rarely, embryonal carcinoma, primary ovarian choriocarcinoma and mixed germ cell tumour.

Ovarian tumours in childhood present with:

- abdominal pain
- an abdominal mass
- urinary frequency
- rectal discomfort
- anorexia.

Treatment involves surgical excision by unilateral oophorectomy with pelvic and para-aortic lymphadenectomy when appropriate. Many tumours also require adjuvant postoperative chemotherapy.

UTERINE TUMOURS

Uterine tumours are extremely rare in childhood and adolescence.

CERVICAL TUMOURS

The most common tumour of the cervix and vagina in girls under 16 years of age is sarcoma botryoides, with 90% of girls presenting before the age of five years.[14] The tumour usually arises from the vagina in young girls and the cervix and upper vagina in older girls or adolescents. The mass is often grape-like in appearance.

The majority of girls (80%) with sarcoma botryoides present with:

- abnormal vaginal bleeding
- bloody vaginal discharge
- a vaginal or abdominal mass.

Diagnosis is made by examination under anaesthesia and biopsy, which should include proctoscopy and cystoscopy. Multimodality treatment combining chemotherapy and radiotherapy with less radical surgery has enabled preservation of reproductive function in early stage disease. Chemotherapy alone with VAC can achieve a 'cure' in 82%.[15]

VAGINAL TUMOURS

Clear-cell adenocarcinoma of the vagina is rare and is associated with vaginal adenosis and exposure to diethylstilboestrol *in utero*. The tumour is usually situated in the upper anterior third of the vagina and may be asymptomatic. However, it often presents with vaginal discharge and/or postcoital bleeding.

Early disease can be treated by wide local excision, lymphadenectomy and adjuvant radiotherapy, whereas more advanced disease requires radical surgery and adjuvant radiotherapy.

VULVAL TUMOURS

Vulval tumours are extremely rare in childhood and adolescence. These include squamous cell carcinoma, malignant melanomas and sarcoma botryoides.

References

1. Curry SL, Schlaerth JB, Kohorn EI, Boyce JB, Gore H, Twiggs LB, et al. Hormonal contraception and trophoblastic sequelae after hydatidiform mole (a Gynecologic Oncology Group study). Am J Obstet Gynecol 1989; 160: 805–11.

2. Bagshawe KD. Risk and prognostic factors in trophoblastic neoplasia. Cancer 1976; 38: 1373–85.

3. Berkowitz RS, Im SS, Bernstein MR, Goldstein DP. Gestational trophoblastic disease: subsequent pregnancy outcome, including repeat molar pregnancy. J Reprod Med 1998; 43: 81–6.

4. Podratz KC, Podczaski ES, Gaffey TA, O'Brien PC, Schray MF, Malkasian GD. Primary carcinoma of the fallopian tube. Am J Obstet Gynecol 1986; 154: 1319–26.

5. Gershenson DM. Management of early ovarian cancer: germ cell and sex-cord stromal tumours. Gynecol Oncol 1994; 55: S62–S72.

6. Gershenson DM. Update on malignant ovarian germ cell tumours. Cancer 1993; 71: 1581–90.

7. O'Connor DM, Norris HJ. The influence of grade on the outcome of stage I ovarian immature (malignant) teratomas and the reproducibility of grading. Int J Gynecol Pathol 1994; 13: 283–9.

8. Segal R, DePetrillo AD, Thomas G. Clinical review of adult granulose cell tumours of the ovary. Gynecol Oncol 1995; 56: 338–44.

9. Rubin SC, Young J, Mikuta JJ. Squamous carcinoma of the vagina: treatment, complications, and long-term follow-up. Gynecol Oncol 1985; 20: 346–53.

10. Benedet JL, Saunders BH. Carcinoma in situ of the vagina. Am J Obstet Gynecol 1984; 148: 695–700.

11. Melnick S, Cole P, Anderson D, Herbst A. Rates and risks of diethylstilboestrol related to clear cell adenocarcinoma of the vagina and cervix. Cancer 1996; 79: 2229-36.

12. Kirkbride P, Fyles A, Rawlings GA, Manchul L, Levin W, Murphy KJ, et al. Carcinoma of the vagina – experience at the Princess Margaret Hospital (1974–1989). Gynecol Oncol 1995; 56: 435–43.

13. Knocke TH, Kucera H, Dotfler D, Pokrajac B, Potter R. Results of post-operative radiotherapy in the treatment of sarcoma of the corpus uteri. Cancer 1998; 83: 1972-9.

14. Copeland LJ, Gershenson DM, Saul PB, Sneige N, Stringer CA, Edwards CL. Sarcoma botryoides of the female genital tract. Obstet Gynecol 1985; 66: 262–6.

15. Raney RB, Crist WM, Maurer HM, Foulkes MA. Prognosis of children with soft tissue sarcoma who relapse after achieving a complete response. Cancer 1983; 52: 44–50.

15 Palliation

Introduction

Approximately 50% of the women who present with a newly diagnosed gynaecological cancer will eventually die as a direct result of their disease. This figure is approximate and will vary geographically as a result of case mix and stage at presentation. Nevertheless, it is a salutary point that palliative effort receives disproportionately less time and study than does our continued efforts to 'cure' patients with gynaecological cancer. This is not to suggest that eradication of disease is not a worthy goal, but a reminder to those charged with the responsibility of managing these patients that part of our work must also be in offering timely and effective palliation. Recognising the differing principles that support curative and palliative intent is fundamental to high quality care in oncology.

Definition

Palliation can be defined as a healthcare strategy directed at alleviating the symptoms of disease without curative intent. Palliation should always be a consideration, although secondary, in patients in whom a curative primary role is planned. A primary palliative attempt, on the other hand, should be focused upon the patient's symptoms and their relief. Some patients may survive many years after such palliative procedures (surgery, radiotherapy and chemotherapy), but long-term survival or even cure is a secondary objective when palliation is the object of the management strategy. Thus:

- curative intent should always have a palliative role as well in symptomatic patients
- palliative intent may have a long-term survival or curative role but this is not the primary objective.

Principles of palliation

Palliation is symptomatically orientated. These symptoms may be physical, such as pain or nausea, or psychological and emotional, such as anxiety and depression. Most, if not all, patients with malignant disease will have a psychological component to their disease and this should not be forgotten.[1,2] Similarly, it is all too easy to interpret a patient's symptom or symptoms in a way that you, the individual clinician sees them. Thus, it might be considered appropriate by a clinician to defunction a woman who has gastrointestinal obstruction associated with vomiting but the patient's major fear and anxiety may be abhorrence of a stoma. Non-surgical palliation may be a better option in this case. The patient requires information that is both understandable and honest if a good palliative result is to be achieved.

Types of palliative approach

Surgery does not always spring to mind as a palliative approach, probably because, in most palliative environments, surgery is a treatment modality that has already been used (with a curative intent) and failed. Secondly, palliative care is multidisciplinary and is not usually surgically led. Physicians and anaesthetists have adopted the primary lead roles here. Finally, surgery is seen to be invasive, traumatic and associated with prolonged recovery intervals. These attributes may seem counter-productive in a woman who has a severely limited life expectancy. A further consideration, and one that is more likely to be considered in cost-conscious health services, is cost efficacy. Can other, less expensive routes achieve the palliative objective?

Radiotherapy and chemotherapy are also useful palliatives but, like surgery, have their shortcomings. Radiotherapy is of huge value, for instance, in palliating pain from bone metastases and may also have some value in treating isolated secondary disease in previously non-irradiated areas. One review has suggested that rapid pain relief can be achieved in up to 70% of patients and last for up to three months.[3] Furthermore, the effect is rapid. Its limitations lie in normal tissue tolerance and the distinct possibility of causing more symptoms than it attempts to alleviate, if used in areas subject to previous irradiation. Chemotherapy, some would argue, is always palliative in the majority of common solid tumours, particularly gynaecological, as cured cases represent the minority. There is also limitation of tolerance, with high toxicity, poor responses in previously heavily treated areas and, of course, the possibility of disturbed renal and marrow function compromising the ability to deliver tumoricidal doses. As in attempts to cure, combinations of treatments may also have a place but less so, given the potential to increase toxicity.

Symptoms

These will depend to a large extent on the site of the disease, whether there are distant metastases and what local involvement has occurred. For example, involvement of the bladder or rectum might provoke functional disturbance of these organs, whereas involvement of the nerve plexuses in the pelvis may cause pain.

The common symptoms associated with gynaecological malignancy are:

- pain
- gastrointestinal problems
- discharge
- incontinence (faecal and urinary)
- psychological and emotional.

Management choices

All treatment modalities can be considered but a balance has to be achieved between the effect of the intervention itself and symptom control. For instance, radiotherapy may lead to almost immediate relief of bone pain, with virtually no morbidity, whereas medical management with opiates may result in excessive drowsiness.

As a good working principle, that which achieves the desired goal with the least morbidity should be considered first and forms the basis of the management plan.

SYMPTOM-SPECIFIC PALLIATION

Palliation should be symptom specific and all of the symptoms need to be considered together. For instance, if a patient had nausea and vomiting due to a high gastrointestinal tract obstruction, a hyperdynamic antiemetic such as metoclopramide might exacerbate the vomiting. Antibiotics can produce nausea and analgesics can cause constipation.

Pain

Pain is one of the most common complaints for which patients seek help. The causes of pain, however, are different in oncology patients. Only about 10% of pain in patients with cancer is caused by non-cancer-related problems; in other words, 90–95% of pain is cancer related. Seventy-five percent relates to pain caused by the cancer, with 15–20% caused by treatments for the disease (i.e. mucositis caused by chemotherapy). Pain is also frequently exacerbated by psychological, emotional and spiritual factors.[4] Patients with cancer-related pain can be categorised into five separate types.

ACUTE CANCER-RELATED PAIN

This is acute pain that may have led to the presentation in the first place, although this is unusual in gynaecological cancers. Pain may also relate to cancer therapies. Such patients' pain may be addressed by therapies directed at the cancer itself, which often provides the most effective and longest lasting relief. These patients usually have good tolerance of their pain psychologically, as they believe that they are likely to respond to treatment and, thus, the pain is unlikely to be protracted.

CHRONIC CANCER-RELATED PAIN

Chronic cancer-associated pain (pain lasting more than three months) is harder to manage. It is usually related to the progression of disease or the long-term sequelae of treatment. The cause is usually obvious and therefore intensive investigation is not necessary. The source of this type of pain can rarely be removed and so treatment is aimed at maximising function and minimising symptoms.

OTHER PAIN CATEGORIES

A third group includes those who, in addition to cancer, also have other conditions that are associated with chronic pain. The fourth group is those who have a history of drug dependence. Both of these groups can require quite complex management and should be managed by specialist pain teams.

The last group are those who are dying and have pain. Here the assessment is done with virtually no laboratory testing and management needs to address all causes of suffering related to dying.

Types of pain

Somatic pain (e.g. arthritis or bone metastases) is constant, dull and aching. It is increased by movement and localised to the area of the lesion. Visceral pain (e.g. myocardial ischaemia, liver metastases) is poorly localised, deep aching or tearing in nature. Neuropathic pain (e.g. sciatica or pelvic nerve-root involvement) is burning and sharp. It is often described as being like an electrical shock.

MEASUREMENT OF PAIN

Pain measurement is subjective and there is a plethora of charts and diaries that can be employed. Some form of assessment is desirable so that management methods that employ graduated or 'ladder'-type application of therapies can be used with reference to some baseline. It also allows for rapid recognition of poor analgesic control with timely dose adjustments.

Management of pain

Pharmacological therapy is the mainstay of cancer pain relief. Satisfactory pain relief can be achieved in over 90% of patients with minimum adverse effects.[5] Oral and transdermal medication will suffice for most. Nonsteroidal anti-inflammatory agents usually will not be effective alone for patients with cancer pain[6] and combination with an opioid will be required for mild to moderate pain. The efficacy of a pain control regimen should be closely and frequently assessed with rapid increase in analgesic power until the pain is controlled.[7] There may be a requirement to address the patient's mental state at the same time, as this will have a powerful influence on the patient's pain threshold. Neuropathic pain may require opioid adjuvants such as tricyclic antidepressants, corticosteroids and/or anticonvulsant.[8] When opioids are used they should always be given with laxatives and some may also generate considerable nausea.

Regional analgesic blocks are also important approaches to pain control. They may be particularly useful when advanced cervical cancer generates nerve root pain.[9]

Gastrointestinal symptoms

NAUSEA AND VOMITING

These symptoms are often amenable to treatment, even if the cause is irreversible. In gynaecological cancer, the most common causes are gastrointestinal obstruction or secondary to chemotherapy. If the underlying cause can be removed then this should certainly be considered and is one of the surgical roles for palliation. Constipation is another common cause of nausea and is often overlooked. Electrolyte imbalance is also a potential cause and should be evaluated, as it may exacerbate bowel obstruction. The approaches to management include simple methods, such as providing frequent small feeds of cold food, removal of foods which the patient finds have an unpleasant odour or appearance and the serving of meals in pleasant and comfortable surroundings.[10]

Pharmacological approaches should take account of whether or not the aetiology of the problem is known (Tables 15.1a and 15.1b).

For patients with gastrointestinal obstruction who are not considered as suitable candidates for surgery, percutaneous gastrostomy may provide relief, particularly in those who have a high level of obstruction.[11] For lower levels of obstruction opioids, scopolamine and haloperidol are usually effective in controlling the nausea, vomiting and pain. Octreotide is also highly effective, as it inhibits gastrointestinal secretions.[12]

Many of these drugs can be administered by slow subcutaneous infusions and this is a particularly attractive route in those intolerant of

Table 15.1a Pharmacological agents for nausea and vomiting when the cause is known

Cause	Agent
Opioid drugs	Prochlorperazine
Delayed gastric emptying	Metoclopramide
Uraemia, liver metastases	Haloperidol, prochlorperazine
Brain metastases	Dexamethasone
Anxiety	Lorazepam
Bowel obstruction	Octreotide

any oral intake. Even in patients who are obstructed and vomiting, small amounts may still be taken by mouth if that is what the patient wishes. Many would prefer to have one or two vomits per day than suffer the problems associated with nasogastric intubation. The latter should ideally be reserved for those recovering from surgical procedures.

ASCITES

Initially, attempts should be made to control ascites with diuretics and appropriate electrolyte supplementation. In refractory cases, paracentesis will be necessary and, if this becomes a frequent requirement, recurrent ascites can be managed by intraperitoneal instillations of fibrotic agents or by the placements of shunts that drain the ascites back into the venous system. Shunts are preferable to repeated paracentesis in those patients who may be expected to live longer than six months.[13,14]

DIARRHOEA

This is less common than constipation and nausea but occurs in 5–10% of end-stage gynaecological cancer patients. The causes include acquired lactose intolerance, drugs, intermittent bowel obstruction, faecal impaction

Table 15.1b Pharmacological agents for nausea and vomiting when the cause is not known

Line of treatment	Agent
Refractory nausea first	Metoclopramide and dexamethasone, plus hydroxazine or diphenhydramine
Second	Ondansetron
	Granisetron
	Haloperidol
Third	Tetrahydrocannabinol

or sphincter compromise. In cervical cancer, another aetiology that should be considered is chronic radiation enteritis. If specific treatment is not available or the cause is unknown, rehydration, avoidance of fats and prescribing loperamide are usually effective. Opioids might be of use if the more simple strategy is not effective.[15]

Vaginal discharge and bleeding

Offensive vaginal discharge and bleeding usually represent a recurrence of tumour at the vaginal vault. Both symptoms are depressing and associated with loss of dignity and reduced mobility. Offensive discharges usually respond well to metronidazole, as the smell is anaerobic in origin. Cautery of vaginal lesions can also be attempted.

Bleeding can be intermittent and chronic and can, in turn, lead to anaemia, which should be corrected. Rest with packing and antibiotics may suffice if the bleeding is not heavy.

Embolisation under radiological control is an effective method of managing bleeding from advanced cervical or other pelvic malignancies as long as a distinct blood supply to the tumour can be identified.[16]

Lymphoedema

Lymphoedema is a consequence both of disease and of surgery, occurring after pelvic and groin node dissection. The lower limb is affected in gynaecological cancers and when severe, may affect mobility (Figure 15.1: plate 15).

When the condition arises as a result of lymphatic metastases, local irradiation to the affected node group might be considered but this is not likely to result in resolution of the problem. Simple measures, such as avoidance of superficial trauma that may cause cellulitis, should be explained to the patient. Elevation of the affected limb in association with massage and graduated pressure stockings can also be of value.

When the condition occurs following lymphadenectomy, the management principles are much the same, although the problem may be anticipated.[17] Patients should be counselled as to the risk prior to lymphadenectomy and the principles of massage and skin care explained. Patients should be referred to a lymphoedema service early. Pressure stockings should only be applied after the post-surgical inflammatory process has subsided, as there is a theoretical risk of increasing the possibility of lymphocyst.

LYMPHOCYST

This is a collection of lymph occurring as a result of obstruction of drainage. Most subside over time and do not require active intervention.

If they become infected they should be treated aggressively with antibiotics. Persisting cysts that are symptomatic or become infected repeatedly should be drained. In the pelvis, they can be marsupialised, allowing free drainage of lymph into the peritoneal cavity (although they not infrequently become reperitonealised).[18] In the groin, drainage should be followed by pressure dressing in an attempt to prevent re-accumulation and encourage fibrosis of the cavity.

Surgery in palliation

Surgery has value largely in four areas:

- to alleviate the symptoms of gastrointestinal tract obstruction
- to remove ureteric obstruction (particularly if the relief of obstructive uropathy results in a return to normal renal function and might allow possible curative chemotherapy to be given. Ureteric stents may be of value in this context. If there is no effective treatment of the cause however, the outcome of surgical relief should be balanced against allowing the patient to die as a result of uraemia)
- to bypass either bowel, urinary tract or both, if they are causing severe fistula related symptoms
- to remove a localised intra-abdominal mass that is causing symptoms.

GASTROINTESTINAL OBSTRUCTION

Gastrointestinal obstruction is usually associated with ovarian cancer. Up to 50% of patients with this disease will have obstruction at some time in their illness. The onset is usually insidious, with repeated admissions for presumed subacute obstruction. Management is non-surgical in the first instance with:

- analgesics
- antispasmodics
- antiemetics
- antibiotics.

Patients should be carefully selected for surgery as not all will derive any benefit. When considering selection for surgery, the causes of the obstruction need to be considered: These include:

- extrinsic pressure
- infiltration of the bowel
- malignant adhesion formation
- peristaltic dysfunction
- mesenteric infiltration.

Table 15.2 Decision making in selecting cases for surgical intervention

Variable	Good surgical candidate	Poor surgical candidate
Initial disease	Localised	Disseminated
Timing of obstruction	> 12 months from completed treatment	< 12 months of completed treatment
Level of obstruction	Low level and single site	High level and/or multiple sites
Imaging	Normal transit of barium through small bowel	Delayed transit of barium
Previous response	Good response to previous treatment	Poor response
Performance status	Good performance status, not malnourished	Poor performance status or malnourished
Previous laparotomies	One previous laparotomy	More than one previous laparotomy
Ascites	Absent	Present
Life expectancy	> 4 months	< 4 months

It is also important to select on the basis of level and number of sites of obstruction.

SELECTING CASES FOR SURGICAL INTERVENTION

After initial management the following criteria are used to select for surgical intervention:

- initial disease status
- timing of obstruction in relation to treatment
- level(s) of obstruction
- imaging findings
- patient's general condition and performance status.

There have been several attempts to develop scoring systems to allow a more objective selection process. None is based on large series of patients and an individual approach is recommended. In general, the features that are of value in making decisions are shown in Table 15.2. It is stressed that these variables should not, as individual variables, influence the final decision. The surgeon must attempt to build a picture of the overall impact of such variables and balance the morbidity and potential success of surgery against the quality of life without surgery.[19]

TYPES OF SURGERY

In ovarian cancer, our most frequent surgical intervention is loop ileostomy. This is a quick procedure, has a rapid recovery, alleviates symptoms associated with large bowel obstruction and, although the stomas can be problematic, in the short-to-medium term this is not so for most patients, given adequate support and stoma care. It is of course essential to ensure that the proximal small bowel is not extensively involved in the disease process.

Resection of bowel may be necessary but if possible avoided because of the risk of anastamotic leak and breakdown in malnourished patients. If there is a solitary metastasis obstructing the bowel and resection and reanastomosis is possible then this should be considered as it obviates the need for a stoma. Side-to-side bypass may also be an alternative if there is widespread disease but only a segment of bowel is involved. The authors have used most of the options in their day-to-day practice and these have included:

- gastrostomy
- jejunostomy
- ileostomy (loop and terminal)
- colostomy (loop transverse, descending and sigmoid)
- end colostomy
- caecostomy
- entero-enterostomy.

If further treatment such as second-line chemotherapy is proposed, this is not strictly a palliative procedure. In effect, surgery is supportive in allowing further attempts at cytoreduction to take place. Nevertheless, it is still aimed at symptom control, which would be a necessary prerequisite to allow further treatment phases.

Surgical approaches to the management of gastrointestinal obstruction are effective in terms of symptom control and allowing early discharge to a home environment, with less dependency and improved self-esteem. In terms of survival, the outcome is not good, although some enjoy a considerable long-term survival. These patients are virtually always those with a solitary circumscribed mass causing bowel dysfunction through external pressure; in other words, they have presented with localised rather than generalised relapse.

Bowel obstruction may also occur in relation to other cancers. Endometrial cancer is similar to ovarian disease, apart from the increased likelihood of more distant disease that may affect the decision for surgical intervention. They may also be older and in far worse general condition than those with ovarian cancer. Despite this, the same principles should apply.

Cervical cancer is different. Localised pelvic disease is more common in comparison to ovarian and endometrial cancer, the patients in general are younger and radiotherapy may already have been used. Large bowel obstruction may be only part of the symptom complex associated with pelvic recurrence. Loop colostomy is often of value however if lower bowel obstruction is the main complaint associated with recurrent cervical cancer. Anastomoses should be avoided in the irradiated patients and the distal portion of bowel should not be occluded.

Fistulae

Fistulae occur when there is loss of integrity between two hollow structures or between a hollow structure and the abdominal wall. They can occur as a result of cancer itself or as a result of surgical or radiotherapeutic intervention. Whatever the cause they are virtually always symptomatic. They are distressing to the patient, often offensive and may lead to excoriation and significant discomfort. The result of these symptoms is a loss of dignity and independence.

Fistulae may affect both urinary and gastrointestinal tracts as part of advanced and incurable disease. Some are iatrogenic, resulting in avascular necrosis following surgery and/or radiotherapy.[20]

LARGE BOWEL FISTULAE

The large bowel may form fistulae with either the vagina (Figure 15.2), bladder or occasionally may be a part of an enterocutaneous fistula. All may result in significant symptoms. Faeculent discharge from the vagina is distressing, can be painful and results in a loss of dignity and independence. Investigation is required to ensure that simple large bowel diversion will result in alleviation of symptoms as occasionally small bowel may also be involved, particularly in the previously irradiated patient. The majority of women with this problem are generally quite well otherwise, and may have a reasonable life expectancy. Colostomy adds significantly to the improved quality of life in these situations.

SMALL BOWEL FISTULAE

Small bowel may become involved in a fistula as a result of malignant infiltration and/or prior irradiation. Although the discharge may be less offensive than a large bowel fistula they can result in significant discomfort because of the volume of loss and the excoriation that usually accompanies exposure to small bowel contents. If there is any doubt as to the source of a fistula, barium studies can be performed or a fistulogram in the case of an enterocutaneous fistula.

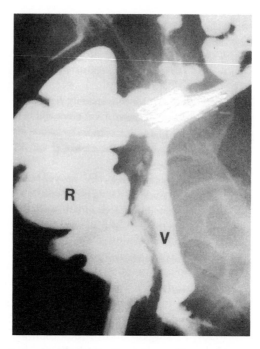

Figure 15.2 Rectovaginal fistulae; R = rectum, V = vagina

When small bowel is involved it is important to determine the highest level involved and take surgical measures to ensure that postoperatively the whole faecal stream is diverted. Fistulae associated with localised pelvic recurrence generally have a longer-term survival than those found in association with widespread intra-abdominal disease. However, there are few nonsurgical modalities that can offer the same degree of palliation as surgery.

ENTEROCUTANEOUS FISTULAE

These are highly distressing and difficult to manage. Tumour that has invaded the anterior abdominal wall or has fungated and involved the bowel usually represents quite advanced intraperitoneal disease. Isolated metastases do occur in the abdominal wall, in wounds and in the track of prior paracenteses. Occasionally they can be managed by placing a colostomy bag over the fistula. This is probably the most appropriate way to manage the situation in women who have a short predicted survival. In other cases it may be necessary to excise the fistula, affected abdominal wall and bowel with a planned bypass or stoma and abdominal wall reconstruction with synthetic mesh.

URINARY FISTULAE

These are most commonly associated with advanced and recurrent cervical cancers. They may be iatrogenic, especially following radiation. Most often they represent malignant disease that has invaded the bladder and interrupted the integrity of the tissues between the bladder and vagina. The condition is easily confirmed by simple clinical examination and passing a urinary catheter and instilling methylene blue dye into the bladder. Occasionally, however, there may be involvement of the ureter and in these situations more detailed investigations are required such as intravenous urogram, cystoscopy and ascending ureterograms. Vesicovaginal fistulae are difficult to manage conservatively, although incontinence pads etc. may provide some relief in the short term. In patients who have a predicted survival in excess of three months, conservative management may lead to deterioration in symptoms and loss of morale and dignity. Furthermore, total urinary incontinence effectively immobilises women. Double balloon catheters are not of much value unless the fistula is small and can be occluded completely by the catheter balloons on either side of the defect.

For vesicovaginal fistula, clinicians are now far more likely to consider urinary diversion. There are problems, in that patients who are malnourished or are already showing signs of renal compromise may not find a very good outcome; similarly, those who have been irradiated run an increased risk of breakdown. Nevertheless, ileal conduits, ureterostomies and occasionally nephrostomy may offer a significant chance of offering good palliation in those judged to require medium- to long-term palliation. External diversion of the urinary stream is preferable to anastomosing the ureters into large bowel as this avoids the notorious biochemical disturbances associated with "wet" colostomies.[21]

Debulking

Significant symptoms might arise purely because of the presence of a mass. This may result in pressure symptoms, abdominal distension and tenesmus. In recurrent vulval cancer, pain, malodour and a significant loss of self-esteem due to the effect on body image may be amenable to debulking.

With regard to recurrent ovarian cancer, large intraperitoneal masses may be amenable to what has become termed salvage surgery.[22,23] In carefully selected symptomatic women, not only can the symptoms associated with the mass be alleviated, but long-term survival has been recorded. Selection is important in order to maximise the chances of resection and avoid operating on those who have widespread and totally unresectable tumour. Even in some of these women, removal of a large mass may provide useful symptomatic relief. Recurrent vulval disease, or occasionally cervical disease, may affect the tissues of the vulva, perineum and groin and provide not only a focus for necrotic fungation and all its accompaniments but also sap the morale of the most stoical of patients. Wide excision of such masses, even with resort to skin grafting, can provide invaluable palliation. It should be remembered that many of these recurrences are slow growing and indolent in nature and without some form of palliation there is likely to be a protracted and miserable end stage to the disease. Radiation might be considered as an alternative in these situations but this can compromise healing if surgery is required at a later date. Conversely, radiation might achieve palliation without recourse to major anatomical distortion or protracted postoperative stay.

SUMMARY

- Palliation is directed at symptom and not disease control.
- Gynaecological oncologists require a commitment to total care.
- Recognition of failed cure should prompt a redefining of management objectives.
- Good palliative care is a team effort.
- Consider all of the symptoms and the patient's emotional state.
- First use treatments with efficacy and low adverse-effect profiles.
- Chemotherapy has a limited role.
- Radiation and surgery have well defined roles in palliation.

References

1. Breitbart W, Bruera E, Chochinov H, Lynch M. Neoropsychiatric syndromes and psychological symptoms in patients with advanced cancer. *J Pain Symptom Manage* 1995; **10**: 131–41.

2. Massie MJ, Popkin MK. Depressive disorders. In: Holland JC, editor. *Psycho-Oncology*. Oxford: Oxford University Press; 1998. p.518–40.

3. Janjan N. Bone metastases: approaches to management. *Semin Oncol* 2001; **4** Suppl 11: 28–34.

4. Foley KM. Pain assessment and cancer pain syndromes. In: Doyle D, Hanks GWC, MacDonald M, editors. *Oxford Textbook of Palliative Medicine*. 2nd ed. Oxford: Oxford University Press; 1997. p.310–30.

5. Jacox A, Carr DB, Payne R. New clinical practice guidelines for the management of pain in patients with cancer. *N Engl J Med* 1994; **330**: 651–5.

6. Eisenberg E, Berkley CS, Carr DB, Mosteller F, Chalmers TC. Efficacy and safety of non-steroidal anti-inflammatory drugs for cancer pain: a meta-analysis. *J Clin Oncol* 1994; **12**: 2756–65.

7. Levy MH. Pharmacologic treatment of cancer pain. *N Engl J Med* 1996; **335**: 1124–32.

8. Portenoy RK. Adjuvant analgesics in pain management. In: Doyle D, Hanks GWC, MacDonald M, editors. *Oxford Textbook of Palliative Medicine*. 2nd ed. Oxford: Oxford University Press; 1997. p.267–81.

9. Du Pen SL, Kharasch ED, Williams A, Peterson DG, Sloan DC, Hasche-Klunder H, *et al*. Chronic epidural bupivacaine-opioid infusion in intractable cancer pain. *Pain* 1992; **49**: 293–300.

10. NCCN. Antiemesis practice guidelines. *Oncology (Huntingt)* 1997; **11**: 57–89.

11. Fainsinger R, Spachynski K, Hanson J, Bruera E. Symptom control in terminally ill patients with malignant bowel obstruction. *J Pain Symptom Manage* 1994; **9**: 12–18.

12. Mercadante S. The role of octreotide in palliative care. *J Pain Symptom Manage* 1994; **9**: 406–11.

13. Faught W, Kirkpatrick JR, Kreport GV, Heymood MS, Lotocki RJ. Peritoneovenous shunt for gynecologic malignant ascites. *J Am Coll Surg* 1995; **180**: 472–4.

14. Soderland C. Denver peritoneovenous shunting for malignant or cirrhotic ascites: a prospective consecutive case series. *Scand J Gastroenterol* 1986; **21**: 1167–72.

15. Mercadante S. Diarrhoea in terminally ill patients: pathophysiology and treatment. *J Pain Symptom Manage* 1995; **10**: 298–309.

16. Mihmanli I, Cantasdemir M, Kantarci F, Halit Yilmaz M, Numan F, Mihmanli V. Percutaneous embolization in the management of intractable vaginal bleeding. *Arch Gynecol Obstet* 2001; **264**: 211–14.

17. Cohen SR, Payne DK, Tunkel RS. Lymphedema: strategies for management. *Cancer* 2001; **92** (4 Suppl): 980–7.

18. Recio FO, Ghamande S, Hempling RE, Piver MS. Effective management of pelvic lymphocysts by laparoscopic marsupialization. *JSLS* 1999; **3(2)**: 97–102.

19. Legendre H, Vanhuyse F, Caroli-Bosc FX, Pector JC. Survival and quality of life after palliative surgery for neoplastic gastrointestinal obstruction. *Eur J Surg Oncol* 2001; **27**: 364–7.

20. Xiang-EW, Shu-mo C, Ya-qin D, Ke W. Treatment of late recurrent vaginal malignancy after initial radiotherapy for carcinoma of the cervix: an analysis of 73 cases. *Gynecol Oncol* 1998; **69**: 125–9.

21. Kochakarn W, Ratana-Olarn K, Viseshsindh V, Muangman V, Gojaseni P. Vesico-vaginal fistula: experience of 230 cases. *J Med Assoc Thailand* 2000; **83**: 1129–32.

22. Gadducci A, Iacconi P, Cosio S, Fanucchi A, Cristofani R, Riccardo Genazzani A. Complete salvage surgical cytoreduction improves further survival of patients with late recurrent ovarian cancer. *Gynecol Oncol* 2000; **79**: 344–9.

23. Garcia AA. Salvage therapy for ovarian cancer. *Curr Oncol Rep* 1999; **1**: 64–70.

Appendix 1
Staging of gynaecological cancers

Staging for carcinoma of the cervix uteri (FIGO 1994)

STAGE 0 Carcinoma *in situ*, cervical intraepithelial neoplasia grade III.

STAGE I Carcinoma confined to the cervix.
Microscopic lesions:
Ia1 Stromal invasion $\leq$ 3 mm, extension $\leq$ 7 mm.
Ia2 Stromal invasion > 3 but $\leq$ 5 mm, extension $\leq$ 7 mm.
Clinically evident lesions:
Ib1 Not greater than 4 cm diameter.
Ib2 Greater than 4 cm.

STAGE II Invasion beyond uterus, but not to pelvic sidewall or lower one-third of the vagina.
IIa No obvious parametrial involvement.
IIb Obvious parametrial involvement.

STAGE III Extension to pelvic sidewall. On rectal examination there is no cancer-free space between tumour and pelvic wall. The tumour involves the lower one-third of the vagina. All cases with hydronephrosis or non-functioning kidney are included, unless due to another cause.
IIIa Involves lower one-third of the vagina. No extension to pelvic sidewall.
IIIb Extension to pelvic sidewall and/or hydronephrosis or non-functioning kidney.

STAGE IV Extension beyond true pelvis or biopsy proven bladder or rectal involvement.
IVa Spread to adjacent organs.
IVb Spread to distant organs.

Staging for carcinoma of the corpus uteri (FIGO 1988)

STAGE I* Confined to the corpus.
Ia Limited to endometrium.
Ib Less than 50% myometrial invasion.
Ic More than 50% myometrial invasion.

Stage II* Cervix involved.
IIa Endocervical glandular involvement only.
IIb Cervical stromal invasion.

Stage III* Spread beyond the corpus not involving rectal or bladder mucosa and not beyond the abdominal cavity.
IIIa Carcinoma involves serosa of uterus or adnexae and/or positive cytology.
IIIb Vaginal involvement.
IIIc Para-aortic/pelvic lymph node involvement.

Stage IV* Bladder or rectal involvement and distant metastases.
IVa Involving bladder or rectal mucosae.
IVb Distant metastases and/or inguinal lymph nodes.

* Cases should be allocated histopathological grades (G):
Gx Grade cannot be assessed.
G1 Well differentiated.
G2 Moderately differentiated.
G3 Poorly/undifferentiated.

Staging for carcinoma of the ovary (FIGO 1988)

Stage I   Growth limited to ovaries.

        Ia   Growth limited to one ovary.

        Ib   Growth limited to both ovaries.

In both **Ia** and **Ib**:

- no ascites.
- no tumour on external surface of ovaries.
- capsule of ovaries must be intact.

    Ic Stage Ia or Ib *with*:

- ascites containing malignant cells *or*
- positive peritoneal washings *or*
- tumour on external surface of one or both ovaries *or*
- capsule ruptured.

Stage II   Growth involving one or both ovaries with pelvic extension.

        IIa   Extension and/or metastases to the uterus or tubes.

        IIb   Extension to other pelvic tissues.

        IIc   Stage IIa or IIb with:

- ascites present containing malignant cells *or*
- positive peritoneal washings.

Stage III   Growth involving one or both ovaries with peritoneal implants outside the pelvis or positive retroperitoneal or inguinal lymph nodes. Superficial liver metastases equals stage III.

        IIIa Tumour grossly limited to the true pelvis with negative nodes, but with histologically confirmed microscopic seeding of abdominal peritoneal surfaces.

        IIIb Tumour with histologically confirmed implants on abdominal peritoneal surfaces none exceeding 2 cm in diameter. Nodes are negative.

        IIIc Abdominal implants greater than 2 cm in diameter or positive retroperitoneal or inguinal lymph nodes.

Stage IV   Growth involving one or both ovaries with distant metastases*.

*If pleural effusion is present there must be positive cytology. Parenchymal liver metastases equals stage IV disease.

Staging for carcinoma of the vulva (FIGO 1996)

(For comparison with TNM [tumour, nodes, metastases] staging, see Chapter 13.)

Stage I   Tumour confined to vulva/perineum no lymph node metastases.

      Ia   Lesions 2 cm or less with stromal invasion 1 mm or less.

      Ib   Lesions 2 cm or less with stromal invasion greater than 1 mm.

Stage II   Tumour confined to vulva/perineum more than 2 cm diameter no lymph node metastases.

Stage III   Tumour of any size arising on the vulva and/or perineum with spread to lower urethra and/or vagina or anus and/or unilateral regional lymph nodes.

Stage IV   Tumour invading bladder, urethra rectum or bone or distant metastases.

      IVa   tumour invading: upper urethra bladder mucosa, rectal mucosa or pelvic bone.
and/or bilateral regional lymph nodes.

      IVb   any distant metastases, including pelvic nodes.

Staging for gestational trophoblastic tumours (FIGO 1991)

Stage I Tumour confined to the uterus.

Stage II Metastasis to the vagina and/or pelvis.

Stage III Metastasis to the lungs.

Stage IV Other distant metastasis with or without lung involvement.

Note: Stages I–IV are subdivided into A–C according to the number of risk factors:
A, without risk factors; B, with one risk factor; C, with two risk factors.

Staging for carcinoma of the fallopian tube (FIGO 1994)

Stage I   Tumour confined to fallopian tubes.

       Ia   Tumour limited to one tube, no serosal penetration, no ascites.

       Ib   Tumour limited to both tubes, no serosal penetration, no ascites.

       Ic   Tumour limited to one or both tubes, with serosal involvement and/or positive ascites or peritoneal washings.

Stage II   Tumour involves one or both fallopian tubes with pelvic extension.

       Ia   Extension and/or metastasis to uterus and/or ovaries.

       IIb   Extension to other pelvic structures.

       IIc   Pelvic extension (IIA or IIB) with positive ascites or peritoneal washings.

Stage III   Tumour involves one or both fallopian tubes, with peritoneal implants outside the pelvis and/or positive regional lymph nodes.

       IIIa   Microscopic peritoneal metastasis outside the pelvis.

       IIIb   Macroscopic peritoneal metastasis outside the pelvis not exceeding 2 cm in size.

       IIIc   Peritoneal metastasis more than 2 cm in size and/or positive regional lymph nodes.

Stage IV   Distant metastasis (excludes peritoneal metastasis).

Staging for carcinoma of the vagina (FIGO 1994)

Stage I   Tumour confined to the vagina.

Stage II   Tumour invades paravaginal tissues but does not extend to pelvic wall.

Stage III   Tumour extends to pelvic wall.

Stage IV   Tumour invades mucosa of bladder or rectum, and/or extends beyond the true pelvis.[a]
                 IVa   Spread to adjacent organs.
                 IVb   Distant metastases.

[a] Note: The presence of bullous oedema is not sufficient evidence to classify a tumour as IVa.

Appendix 2
Emergencies in gynaecological oncology and complications of treatment

Introduction

Gynaecological malignancies include ovarian, tubal, uterine, cervical, vaginal and vulval cancers. These tumours may present as an emergency with abnormal bleeding, pain and disordered bowel or bladder function or as a pelvic or genital mass.

The surgical and non-surgical treatments of gynaecological malignancies are associated with complications, which may also present as an emergency. The emergency presentations and management specific to each tumour site are discussed below.

Ovarian cancer

EMERGENCY PRESENTATION

Many patients present with vague gastrointestinal symptoms, urinary frequency and/or urgency or a pelvic abdominal mass. In advanced disease they can present as an emergency with:

- **abdominal pain** due to torsion or infarction of the tumour or due to obstruction of an intra-abdominal viscus
- **rapid abdominal distension** due to tumour growth or ascites
- **partial or total bowel obstruction** due to extrinsic pressure on the bowel, infiltration of the mesenteries and/or a direct toxic effect decreasing bowel activity
- **urinary tract obstruction** due to ureteric obstruction
- **uterovaginal prolapse** due to the increased intra-abdominal pressure
- **cardiorespiratory compromise** due to gross ascites or pleural effusion.

INVESTIGATIONS

- Routine preoperative tests required for any laparotomy for suspected gynaecological malignancy:
  - full blood count
  - U&Es
  - liver function tests
  - chest X-ray (see also Chapter 4)
- CT scan of the pelvis/abdomen may be useful to delineate the tumour.
- Serum CA 125 levels
- βhCG, AFP, carcinoembryonic antigen – if the patient is young and a germ cell tumour is suspected.

TREATMENT

Primary debulking or cytoreductive surgery

The aim is to perform accurate staging of the disease and total macroscopic

Table A2.1 Complications of laparotomy for gynaecological malignancy

Complication	Causes/treatment
Intraoperative	
Haemorrhage	Especially from the infundibulopelvic ligaments or the bed of an incompletely resected pelvic tumour, which may require direct pressure, the use of a haemostatic substance e.g. Surgicell®, or even internal iliac artery ligation
Bowel damage	Due to direct tumour involvement or adhesion formation
Ureteric or bladder damage	Due to close proximity to tumour or tumour spread
Damage to large blood vessels	Compression or infiltration of external iliac arteries and veins
Direct trauma to other intra-abdominal organs	On resection of metastases or due to retraction
Postoperative Ileus	Intraoperative nasogastric tube insertion is advised
Wound dehiscence or incisional hernia	Mass closure is advised
Wound infection	Give prophylactic antibiotics
Deep vein thrombosis and pulmonary embolism	Decrease risk by adequate hydration, thromboembolic deterrent stockings, thromboprophylaxis and early mobilisation

Table A2.2 Complications of chemotherapy

System affected	Complication	Comments/treatment
Haematological	Myelosuppression (in common with carboplatin):	
	Granulocytopenia	Predisposing to sepsis; use prophylactic, broad-spectrum antibiotics in febrile granulocytopenic patients
	Thrombocytopenia	With a risk of spontaneous haemorrhage
	Anaemia	Usually presents after several courses of chemotherapy
Gastrointestinal	Nausea and vomiting	Common adverse effects. 5-HT$_3$ antagonists are effective treatment
	Mucositis	Mouth and pharyngeal ulceration, oesophagitis causing dysphagia, bowel ulceration resulting in diarrhoea or necrotising enterocolitis (NEC) in severe cases with granulocytopenia. Treatment is with intravenous hydration, electrolyte replacement, antimotility drugs e.g. codeine phosphate and vancomycin in NEC
Genitourinary	Acute renal failure	Cisplatin, particularly, causes dose-related renal tubular toxicity. Pre- and post-treatment intravenous hydration is used
	Haemorrhagic cystitis	Due to the irritant effect on the bladder mucosa of acrolein, the toxic metabolite of cyclophosphamide. Hydration, diuresis and mesna (sodium mercaptoethane sulfonate) help to prevent this
Hepatotoxicity	Elevation of liver enzymes may occur	
Neurotoxicity		Many cytotoxic drugs cause some central or peripheral neurotoxicity
Cisplatin	Ototoxicity, peripheral neuropathy, and, rarely, retrobulbar neuritis and blindness	
Paclitaxel	Associated with peripheral sensory neuropathy	Neurotoxicity increased with combination cisplatin therapy
Immunosuppression	Suppression of cellular and humoral immunity	Predisposes to opportunistic infection

Hypersensitivity reactions		Associated with carboplatin, paclitaxel and anaphylaxis with cisplatin
Alopecia		Usually reversible, common with paclitaxel; associated with significant psychological morbidity
Gonadal dysfunction	Infertility	Many cytotoxics cause infertility. Successful pregnancies have been achieved after cisplatin-based chemotherapy
	Teratogenicity	All cytotoxics carry this risk
Second malignancies		Cisplatin is associated with the development of acute leukaemia

clearance. Minimal residual disease is achieved if no tumour mass greater than 1 cm^3 is left. In the majority of cases, temporary supportive treatment can be instituted to allow for a proper preoperative assessment and elective surgery at a time when the gynaecological oncology team is available. If surgery has to be performed as an emergency then the

Table A2.3   Complications of radiotherapy

System/organ affected	Complications
Acute	
Skin	Erythema or desquamation
Bowels	Diarrhoea
Bladder	Irritability, frequency and dysuria
Bone marrow suppression	Anaemia, thrombocytopenia, neutropenia
Late	
Small bowel	Subacute or acute obstruction, bleeding, perforation, fistulae, malabsorption
Large bowel	Proctosigmoiditis, rectovaginal fistula and rectosigmoid obstruction, stricture, perforation or fistulous communication with other intra-abdominal organs
Bladder	Contracture with reduced capacity, haemorrhagic cystitis, vesicovaginal fistula, ureteric obstruction and hydronephrosis
Ovarian failure	
Vaginal atrophy and stenosis	

gynaecological cancer team should be informed and the surgical principles that pertain in an elective situation should be applied. If the patient is unable to withstand major surgery then the minimum required to provide short-term support should be done and a more radical elective procedure performed when the patient is fit. The type of surgery is described in more detail in Chapter 5.

The complications of primary debulking surgery are common to all laparotomies performed for gynaecological malignancy (see Table A2.1).

Chemotherapy
Patients with advanced disease (stage II–IV) should receive adjuvant chemotherapy. Paclitaxel in combination with a platinum therapy (cisplatin or carboplatin) should be the standard initial adjuvant therapy. The evidence for this is detailed in Chapter 10.

There is no overall survival benefit obtained from adjuvant chemotherapy in patients with stage Ia or Ib disease with well- or moderately-differentiated tumours. Paclitaxel/platinum combination chemotherapy is also recommended in the treatment of recurrent (or resistant) ovarian cancer if the patient has not previously received this drug combination.

The complications of chemotherapy are listed in Table A2.2.

Endometrial carcinoma

PRESENTATION

Endometrial carcinoma rarely presents as an emergency although occasionally postmenopausal bleeding can be very profuse and prompt emergency referral. Other presenting symptoms include:

- abdominal pain
- pelvic mass due to enlarged uterus
- pyometra: bloody vaginal discharge due to obstruction of the lower uterine cavity which becomes distended with infected secretions
- abnormal glandular cytology or endometrial cells on cervical cytology.

MANAGEMENT

In an emergency situation the primary objective is to provide supportive care and stabilise the situation. This may require transfusion and occasionally an emergency hysterectomy.

In women who are unfit for surgery, bleeding may be brought under control by pelvic radiotherapy. The complications of radiotherapy are shown in Table A2.3.

Vaginal hysterectomy or laparoscopically assisted vaginal hysterectomy can be considered in patients with marked obesity or medical problems placing them at high risk of complications from abdominal surgery. Complications of vaginal hysterectomy include:

- vaginal bleeding: requiring suturing of the vaginal vault
- intra-abdominal bleeding: bleeding from a pedicle requiring laparotomy
- infected vault haematoma: often settle with antibiotics, but may require surgical drainage.

Cervical cancer

It is unusual for cervical cancer to present as an emergency. When it does, bleeding and pain are the most likely presenting symptoms. Rarely, renal failure may be the first presenting symptom although it is usually possible to elicit a history highly suggestive of carcinoma that predates the emergency presentation by several months.

PRESENTATION

Cervical carcinoma often presents early with:

- abnormal vaginal bleeding: postcoital, intermenstrual or postmenopausal. Bleeding be haemorrhagic requiring resuscitation, vaginal packing and rarely, pelvic irradiation or emergency surgery
- vaginal discharge, often bloodstained
- abnormal cervical cytology: detection on subsequent colposcopy.

Late disease presents with:

- malodorous vaginal discharge: infection of tumour bulk with anaerobes
- pelvic pain due to infiltration of the pelvic sidewalls
- referred leg pain due to invasion of the lumbrosacral plexus
- bowel or bladder disturbance: constipation, tenesmus, rectal bleeding, urinary frequency, haematuria or vaginal passage of urine or faeces if a fistula is present
- pelvic mass, in advanced disease
- vesicovaginal and/or rectovaginal fistulae.

INVESTIGATIONS AND STAGING

See Appendix 1 for full details of FIGO staging. A cervical tumour mass is usually visible either macroscopically or colposcopically. If cervical cancer is suspected in an emergency setting, a biopsy can usually be taken without recourse to general anaesthesia. It is not a substitute for formal staging but allows a diagnosis to be made while the patient is stabilised.

Table A2.4 Complications of surgical treatment for cervical cancer

Stage	Treatment	Complications
Ia1	LLETZ Knife cone biopsy	Secondary haemorrhage, due to infection, is treated with bed rest, antibiotics and, rarely, cervical suturing
	Simple hysterectomy	Complications as for laparotomy
Ia2	Knife cone biopsy Wertheim's hysterectomy and lymph node dissection	See Table A2.1 for complications
	Radical trachelectomy	Vaginal procedure with excision of cervix, upper vagina and parametrium (uterine body is left in situ); immediate complications are infection and bleeding
Ib1	Wertheim's hysterectomy and lymph node dissection	See Table A2.1 for complications
Ib2	Preoperative chemoradiation and adjuvant hysterectomy	
IIa	Schauta radical vaginal hysterectomy and lymph node dissection	Involves taking a vaginal cuff, often with enlargement of the vaginal orifice with a Schuchardt's incision (like a large mediolateral episiotomy); decreased operative mortality, c.f. Wertheim's, complications as that for vaginal hysterectomy with increased risk of ureteric damage

TREATMENT

Bleeding can usually be controlled temporarily by vaginal packing with concurrent antibiotics. The latter are required, as secondary infection is one cause of haemorrhage. Blood transfusion may be necessary and even if the bleeding is not profuse, raising the haemoglobin may have treatment effects by enhancing the effect of radiotherapy. Pain should be managed aggressively as part of the initial stabilisation and assessment process. In a minority of situations, haemorrhage is severe and may necessitate additional control measures such as selective embolisation. Once the patient has been stabilised, management follows the pathway for cases presenting in a non-emergency fashion (see Chapters 5 and 12 for full details). Complications of surgical treatment for cervical cancer are given in Table A2.4. Complications of Wertheim hysterectomy and lymph node dissection are as for laparotomy. Haemorrhage occurs at these sites:

- ureteric tunnel
- paracolpos and vaginal edge
- external iliac artery and vein
- obturator fossa
- bifurcation of common iliac artery and vein
- para-aortic lymph nodes (the use of regional anaesthesia reduces small vessel oozing).

Ureteric dysfunction occurs due to:

- damage to the ureteric blood supply
- damage to the ureteric nerve supply
- oedema of the wall of the ureter
- periureteric infection in the retroperitoneal space.

Ureteric stricture and ureterovaginal fistulae develop as late complications and may require surgery. Bladder dysfunction occurs due to:

- damage to sympathetic nerves in uterosacral and cardinal ligaments results in bladder hypertonicity due to parasympathetics
- oedema of bladder neck and muscle
- hypotonicity as a result of overdistension of a hypertonic bladder (catherisation for six to eight days postoperatively is recommended).

Other complications include:

- urinary tract infection
- vesicovaginal fistulae
- pelvic lymphocysts of the pelvic brim or pelvic sidewall can cause pain, obstruction or become infected; they may require surgical drainage
- peripheral leg lymphoedema may develop late and require specialised massage
- nerve damage to the obturator, genitofemoral, femoral, perineal or sciatic nerves
- sexual dysfunction: this is increased if patient receives adjuvant radiotherapy.

Vulval cancer

PRESENTATION

When presenting as an emergency, the usual symptoms will be pain (often resulting in the inability of the patient to sit comfortably), bleeding and urinary retention. Delay in presentation is not unusual in cancer of the vulva, therefore quite advanced disease can present in the emergency situation. As with the other cancers considered in this section, the principles of management remain the same. The patient should be stabilised if necessary, symptom control instituted and then the patient should be assessed and managed as with non-emergency presentation.

In advanced or recurrent disease the groins may be involved with tumour. This raises the possibility of infiltration and rupture of the vessels in the groin. This is a terminal event in vulval cancer. If this occurs, morphine should be administered intravenously to sedate the patient who will be agitated and anxious, packs may be applied to the bleeding area but the excessive haemorrhage inevitably leads to circulatory failure.

The assessment and management of vulval cancer is discussed in Chapter 13.

PLATE 1

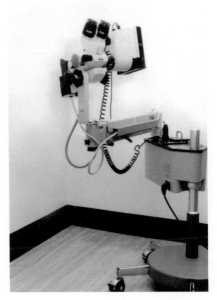

Figure 3.2 Colposcope

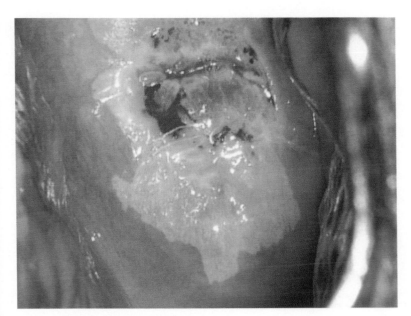

Figure 3.3 Acetowhite epithelium

PLATE 2

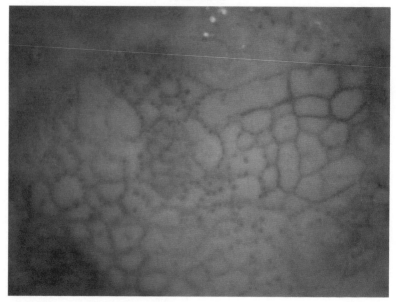

Figure 3.4a Mosaic and punctation

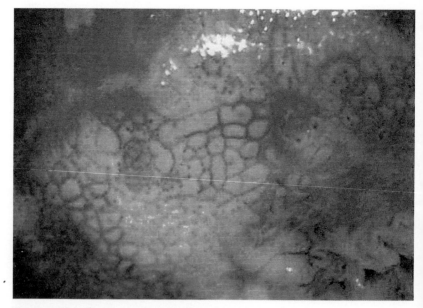

Figure 3.4b Mosaic and punctation

PLATE 3

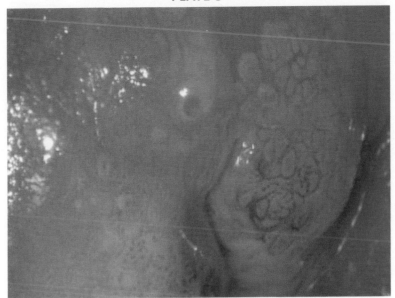

Figure 3.5 Punctation

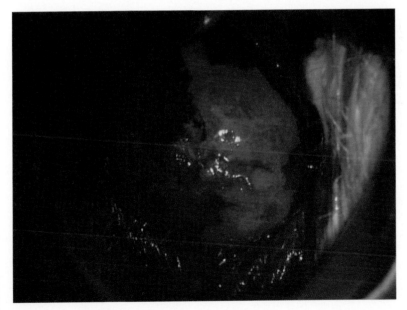

Figure 3.6 Schiller's test

PLATE 4

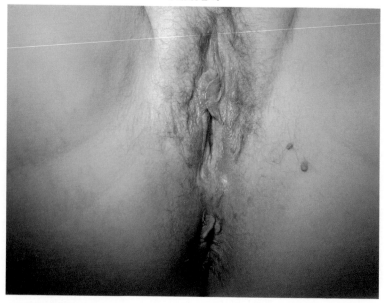

Figure 3.8 Multifocal VIN

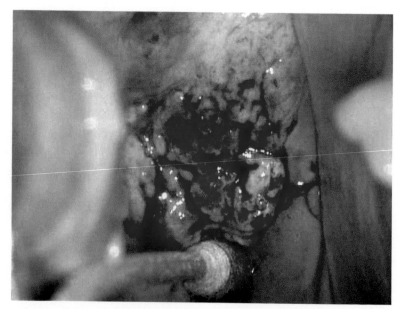

Figure 4.1 Cervical cancer presenting with postcoital bleeding

PLATE 5

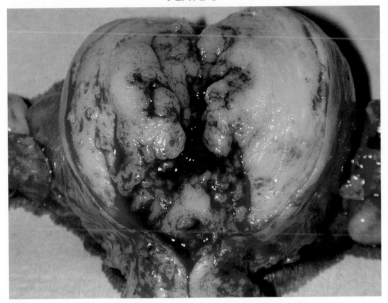

Figure 4.3 Endometrial cancer showing myometrial penetration

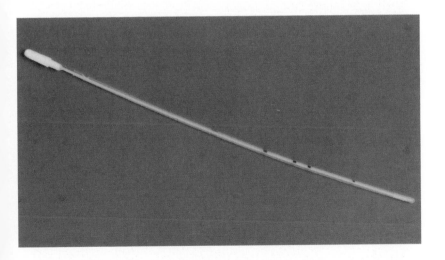

Figure 4.4 Pipelle endometrial sampler

PLATE 6

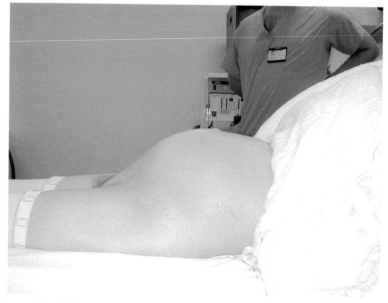

Figure 4.5 Malignant ascites pre-operatively

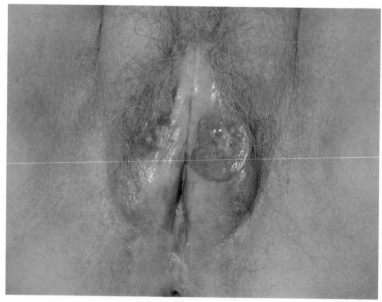

Figure 4.7 Vulval cancer arising in lichen sclerosus

PLATE 7

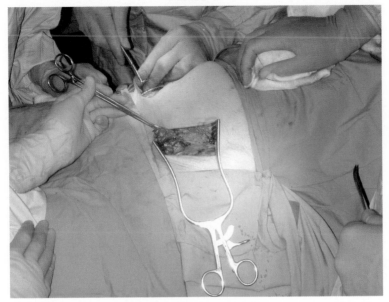

Figure 5.3 Vulval cancer separate groin incisions

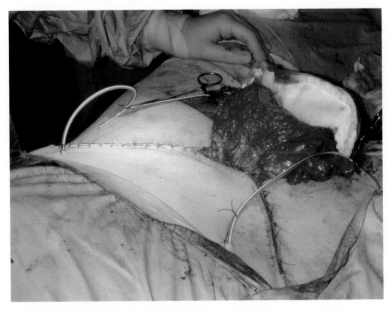

Figure 5.4 En-bloc radical vulvectomy

PLATE 8

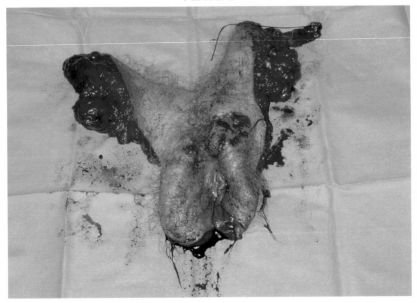

Figure 5.5 En-bloc radical vulvectomy specimen

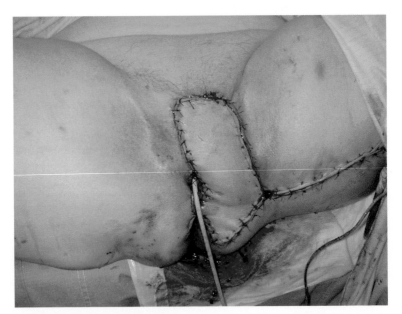

Figure 5.6 Simple rotational flap

PLATE 9

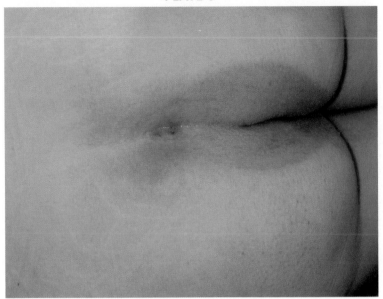

Figure 7.1 Skin erythema reaction post-radiotherapy

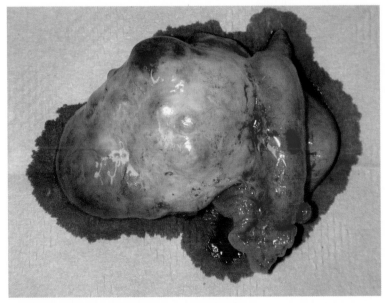

Figure 10.1 Intact malignant ovarian cyst stage 1

PLATE 10

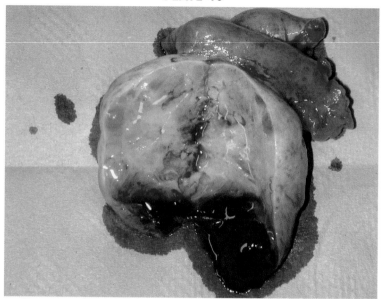

Figure 10.2 Same cyst shown in Figure 10.3 opened showing solid components

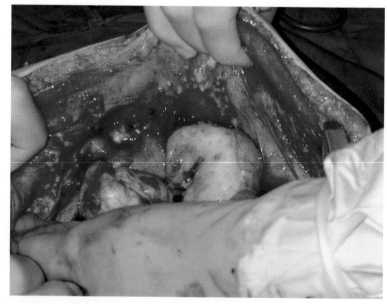

Figure 10.3 Advanced ovarian tumour with seedlings

PLATE 11

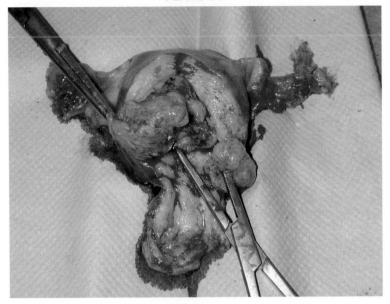

Figure 11.3 Endometrial cancer superficially invasive

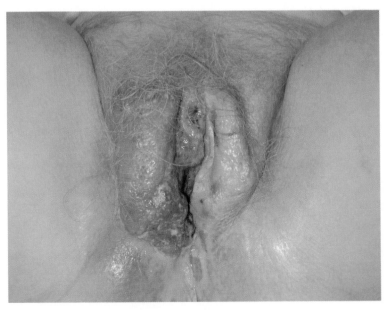

Figure 13.1 Diagnostic wedge biopsy of vulva

PLATE 12

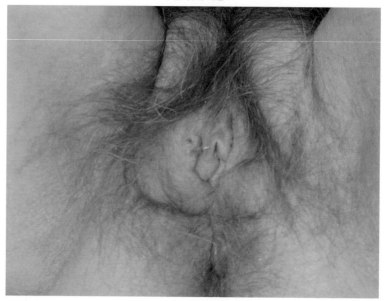

Figure 13.2 Excision biopsy of small vulval lesion

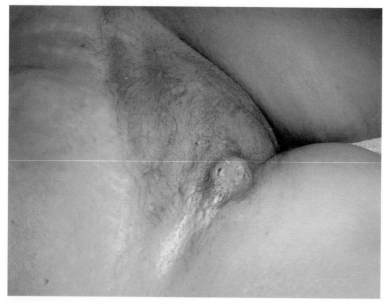

Figure 13.4 Fungating right groin node

PLATE 13

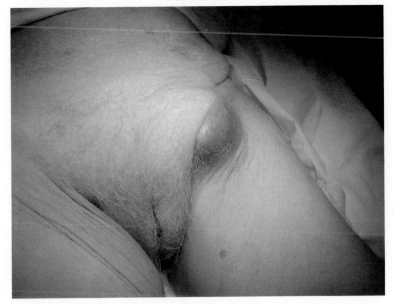

Figure 13.5 Enlarged malignant left groin node

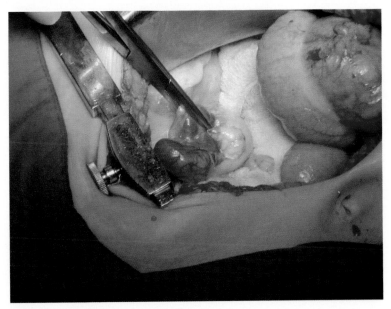

Figure 14.1 Left fallopian tube cancer

PLATE 14

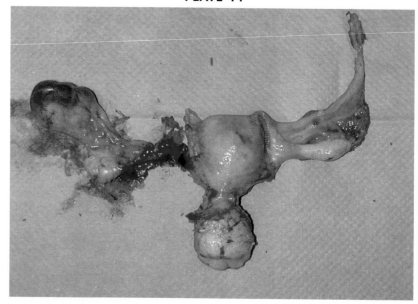

Figure 14.2 Hysterectomy specimen showing normal ovaries

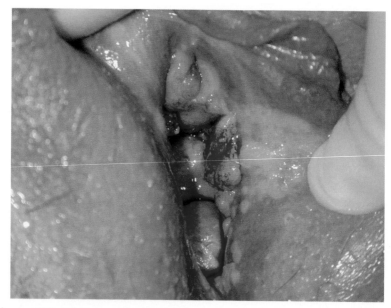

Figure 14.3 Primary vaginal cancer

PLATE 15

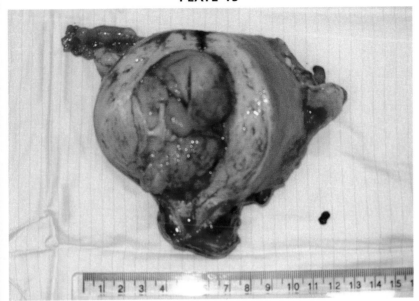

Figure 14.4 Mixed müllerian tumour

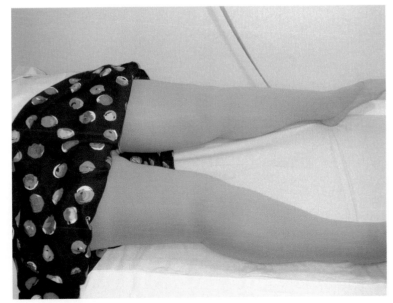

Figure 15.1 Lymphoedema

Appendix 1
Staging of gynaecological cancers

Staging for carcinoma of the cervix uteri (FIGO 1994)

STAGE 0 Carcinoma *in situ*, cervical intraepithelial neoplasia grade III.

STAGE I Carcinoma confined to the cervix.
Microscopic lesions:
Ia1 Stromal invasion $\leq$ 3 mm, extension $\leq$ 7 mm.
Ia2 Stromal invasion > 3 but $\leq$ 5 mm, extension $\leq$ 7 mm.
Clinically evident lesions:
Ib1 Not greater than 4 cm diameter.
Ib2 Greater than 4 cm.

STAGE II Invasion beyond uterus, but not to pelvic sidewall or lower one-third of the vagina.
IIa No obvious parametrial involvement.
IIb Obvious parametrial involvement.

STAGE III Extension to pelvic sidewall. On rectal examination there is no cancer-free space between tumour and pelvic wall. The tumour involves the lower one-third of the vagina. All cases with hydronephrosis or non-functioning kidney are included, unless due to another cause.
IIIa Involves lower one-third of the vagina. No extension to pelvic sidewall.
IIIb Extension to pelvic sidewall and/or hydronephrosis or non-functioning kidney.

STAGE IV Extension beyond true pelvis or biopsy proven bladder or rectal involvement.
IVa Spread to adjacent organs.
IVb Spread to distant organs.

Staging for carcinoma of the corpus uteri (FIGO 1988)

STAGE I* Confined to the corpus.
- **Ia** Limited to endometrium.
- **Ib** Less than 50% myometrial invasion.
- **Ic** More than 50% myometrial invasion.

Stage II* Cervix involved.
- **IIa** Endocervical glandular involvement only.
- **IIb** Cervical stromal invasion.

Stage III* Spread beyond the corpus not involving rectal or bladder mucosa and not beyond the abdominal cavity.
- **IIIa** Carcinoma involves serosa of uterus or adnexae and/or positive cytology.
- **IIIb** Vaginal involvement.
- **IIIc** Para-aortic/pelvic lymph node involvement.

Stage IV* Bladder or rectal involvement and distant metastases.
- **IVa** Involving bladder or rectal mucosae.
- **IVb** Distant metastases and/or inguinal lymph nodes.

* Cases should be allocated histopathological grades (G):
- **Gx** Grade cannot be assessed.
- **G1** Well differentiated.
- **G2** Moderately differentiated.
- **G3** Poorly/undifferentiated.

Staging for carcinoma of the ovary (FIGO 1988)

Stage I Growth limited to ovaries.

    Ia Growth limited to one ovary.

    Ib Growth limited to both ovaries.

In both **Ia** and **Ib**:

- no ascites.
- no tumour on external surface of ovaries.
- capsule of ovaries must be intact.

    Ic Stage Ia or Ib *with*:
- ascites containing malignant cells *or*
- positive peritoneal washings *or*
- tumour on external surface of one or both ovaries *or*
- capsule ruptured.

Stage II Growth involving one or both ovaries with pelvic extension.

    IIa Extension and/or metastases to the uterus or tubes.

    IIb Extension to other pelvic tissues.

    IIc Stage IIa or IIb with:
- ascites present containing malignant cells *or*
- positive peritoneal washings.

Stage III Growth involving one or both ovaries with peritoneal implants outside the pelvis or positive retroperitoneal or inguinal lymph nodes. Superficial liver metastases equals stage III.

    IIIa Tumour grossly limited to the true pelvis with negative nodes, but with histologically confirmed microscopic seeding of abdominal peritoneal surfaces.

    IIIb Tumour with histologically confirmed implants on abdominal peritoneal surfaces none exceeding 2 cm in diameter. Nodes are negative.

    IIIc Abdominal implants greater than 2 cm in diameter or positive retroperitoneal or inguinal lymph nodes.

Stage IV Growth involving one or both ovaries with distant metastases*.

*If pleural effusion is present there must be positive cytology. Parenchymal liver metastases equals stage IV disease.

Staging for carcinoma of the vulva (FIGO 1996)

(For comparison with TNM [tumour, nodes, metastases] staging, see Chapter 13.)

Stage I   Tumour confined to vulva/perineum no lymph node metastases.
   Ia   Lesions 2 cm or less with stromal invasion 1 mm or less.
   Ib   Lesions 2 cm or less with stromal invasion greater than 1 mm.

Stage II   Tumour confined to vulva/perineum more than 2 cm diameter no lymph node metastases.

Stage III   Tumour of any size arising on the vulva and/or perineum with spread to lower urethra and/or vagina or anus and/or unilateral regional lymph nodes.

Stage IV   Tumour invading bladder, urethra rectum or bone or distant metastases.
   IVa   tumour invading: upper urethra bladder mucosa, rectal mucosa or pelvic bone.
   and/or bilateral regional lymph nodes.
   IVb   any distant metastases, including pelvic nodes.

Staging for gestational trophoblastic tumours (FIGO 1991)

Stage I   Tumour confined to the uterus.

Stage II   Metastasis to the vagina and/or pelvis.

Stage III Metastasis to the lungs.

Stage IV   Other distant metastasis with or without lung involvement.

Note: Stages I–IV are subdivided into A–C according to the number of risk factors:
A, without risk factors; B, with one risk factor; C, with two risk factors.

Staging for carcinoma of the fallopian tube (FIGO 1994)

Stage I   Tumour confined to fallopian tubes.
  - **Ia** Tumour limited to one tube, no serosal penetration, no ascites.
  - **Ib** Tumour limited to both tubes, no serosal penetration, no ascites.
  - **Ic** Tumour limited to one or both tubes, with serosal involvement and/or positive ascites or peritoneal washings.

Stage II   Tumour involves one or both fallopian tubes with pelvic extension.
  - **Ia** Extension and/or metastasis to uterus and/or ovaries.
  - **IIb** Extension to other pelvic structures.
  - **IIc** Pelvic extension (IIA or IIB) with positive ascites or peritoneal washings.

Stage III   Tumour involves one or both fallopian tubes, with peritoneal implants outside the pelvis and/or positive regional lymph nodes.
  - **IIIa** Microscopic peritoneal metastasis outside the pelvis.
  - **IIIb** Macroscopic peritoneal metastasis outside the pelvis not exceeding 2 cm in size.
  - **IIIc** Peritoneal metastasis more than 2 cm in size and/or positive regional lymph nodes.

Stage IV   Distant metastasis (excludes peritoneal metastasis).

Staging for carcinoma of the vagina (FIGO 1994)

Stage I   Tumour confined to the vagina.

Stage II   Tumour invades paravaginal tissues but does not extend to pelvic wall.

Stage III Tumour extends to pelvic wall.

Stage IV   Tumour invades mucosa of bladder or rectum, and/or extends beyond the true pelvis.[a]
IVa Spread to adjacent organs.
IVb Distant metastases.

[a] Note: The presence of bullous oedema is not sufficient evidence to classify a tumour as IVa.

Appendix 2 Emergencies in gynaecological oncology and complications of treatment

Introduction

Gynaecological malignancies include ovarian, tubal, uterine, cervical, vaginal and vulval cancers. These tumours may present as an emergency with abnormal bleeding, pain and disordered bowel or bladder function or as a pelvic or genital mass.

The surgical and non-surgical treatments of gynaecological malignancies are associated with complications, which may also present as an emergency. The emergency presentations and management specific to each tumour site are discussed below.

Ovarian cancer

EMERGENCY PRESENTATION

Many patients present with vague gastrointestinal symptoms, urinary frequency and/or urgency or a pelvic abdominal mass. In advanced disease they can present as an emergency with:

- **abdominal pain** due to torsion or infarction of the tumour or due to obstruction of an intra-abdominal viscus
- **rapid abdominal distension** due to tumour growth or ascites
- **partial or total bowel obstruction** due to extrinsic pressure on the bowel, infiltration of the mesenteries and/or a direct toxic effect decreasing bowel activity
- **urinary tract obstruction** due to ureteric obstruction
- **uterovaginal prolapse** due to the increased intra-abdominal pressure
- **cardiorespiratory compromise** due to gross ascites or pleural effusion.

INVESTIGATIONS

- Routine preoperative tests required for any laparotomy for suspected gynaecological malignancy:
  - full blood count
  - U&Es
  - liver function tests
  - chest X-ray (see also Chapter 4)
- CT scan of the pelvis/abdomen may be useful to delineate the tumour.
- Serum CA 125 levels
- βhCG, AFP, carcinoembryonic antigen – if the patient is young and a germ cell tumour is suspected.

TREATMENT

Primary debulking or cytoreductive surgery

The aim is to perform accurate staging of the disease and total macroscopic

Table A2.1 Complications of laparotomy for gynaecological malignancy

Complication	Causes/treatment
Intraoperative	
Haemorrhage	Especially from the infundibulopelvic ligaments or the bed of an incompletely resected pelvic tumour, which may require direct pressure, the use of a haemostatic substance e.g. Surgicell®, or even internal iliac artery ligation
Bowel damage	Due to direct tumour involvement or adhesion formation
Ureteric or bladder damage	Due to close proximity to tumour or tumour spread
Damage to large blood vessels	Compression or infiltration of external iliac arteries and veins
Direct trauma to other intra-abdominal organs	On resection of metastases or due to retraction
Postoperative Ileus	Intraoperative nasogastric tube insertion is advised
Wound dehiscence or incisional hernia	Mass closure is advised
Wound infection	Give prophylactic antibiotics
Deep vein thrombosis and pulmonary embolism	Decrease risk by adequate hydration, thromboembolic deterrent stockings, thromboprophylaxis and early mobilisation

Table A2.2 Complications of chemotherapy

System affected	Complication	Comments/treatment
Haematological	Myelosuppression (in common with carboplatin):	
	Granulocytopenia	Predisposing to sepsis; use prophylactic, broad-spectrum antibiotics in febrile granulocytopenic patients
	Thrombocytopenia	With a risk of spontaneous haemorrhage
	Anaemia	Usually presents after several courses of chemotherapy
Gastrointestinal	Nausea and vomiting	Common adverse effects. $5\text{-}HT_3$ antagonists are effective treatment
	Mucositis	Mouth and pharyngeal ulceration, oesophagitis causing dysphagia, bowel ulceration resulting in diarrhoea or necrotising enterocolitis (NEC) in severe cases with granulocytopenia. Treatment is with intravenous hydration, electrolyte replacement, antimotility drugs e.g. codeine phosphate and vancomycin in NEC
Genitourinary	Acute renal failure	Cisplatin, particularly, causes dose-related renal tubular toxicity. Pre- and post-treatment intravenous hydration is used
	Haemorrhagic cystitis	Due to the irritant effect on the bladder mucosa of acrolein, the toxic metabolite of cyclophosphamide. Hydration, diuresis and mesna (sodium mercaptoethane sulfonate) help to prevent this
Hepatotoxicity	Elevation of liver enzymes may occur	
Neurotoxicity		Many cytotoxic drugs cause some central or peripheral neurotoxicity
Cisplatin	Ototoxicity, peripheral neuropathy, and, rarely, retrobulbar neuritis and blindness	
Paclitaxel	Associated with peripheral sensory neuropathy	Neurotoxicity increased with combination cisplatin therapy
Immunosuppression	Suppression of cellular and humoral immunity	Predisposes to opportunistic infection

Hypersensitivity reactions		Associated with carboplatin, paclitaxel and anaphylaxis with cisplatin
Alopecia		Usually reversible, common with paclitaxel; associated with significant psychological morbidity
Gonadal dysfunction	Infertility	Many cytotoxics cause infertility. Successful pregnancies have been achieved after cisplatin-based chemotherapy
	Teratogenicity	All cytotoxics carry this risk
Second malignancies		Cisplatin is associated with the development of acute leukaemia

clearance. Minimal residual disease is achieved if no tumour mass greater than 1 cm^3 is left. In the majority of cases, temporary supportive treatment can be instituted to allow for a proper preoperative assessment and elective surgery at a time when the gynaecological oncology team is available. If surgery has to be performed as an emergency then the

Table A2.3   Complications of radiotherapy

System/organ affected	Complications
Acute	
Skin	Erythema or desquamation
Bowels	Diarrhoea
Bladder	Irritability, frequency and dysuria
Bone marrow suppression	Anaemia, thrombocytopenia, neutropenia
Late	
Small bowel	Subacute or acute obstruction, bleeding, perforation, fistulae, malabsorption
Large bowel	Proctosigmoiditis, rectovaginal fistula and rectosigmoid obstruction, stricture, perforation or fistulous communication with other intra-abdominal organs
Bladder	Contracture with reduced capacity, haemorrhagic cystitis, vesicovaginal fistula, ureteric obstruction and hydronephrosis
Ovarian failure	
Vaginal atrophy and stenosis	

gynaecological cancer team should be informed and the surgical principles that pertain in an elective situation should be applied. If the patient is unable to withstand major surgery then the minimum required to provide short-term support should be done and a more radical elective procedure performed when the patient is fit. The type of surgery is described in more detail in Chapter 5.

The complications of primary debulking surgery are common to all laparotomies performed for gynaecological malignancy (see Table A2.1).

Chemotherapy

Patients with advanced disease (stage II–IV) should receive adjuvant chemotherapy. Paclitaxel in combination with a platinum therapy (cisplatin or carboplatin) should be the standard initial adjuvant therapy. The evidence for this is detailed in Chapter 10.

There is no overall survival benefit obtained from adjuvant chemotherapy in patients with stage Ia or Ib disease with well- or moderately-differentiated tumours. Paclitaxel/platinum combination chemotherapy is also recommended in the treatment of recurrent (or resistant) ovarian cancer if the patient has not previously received this drug combination.

The complications of chemotherapy are listed in Table A2.2.

Endometrial carcinoma

PRESENTATION

Endometrial carcinoma rarely presents as an emergency although occasionally postmenopausal bleeding can be very profuse and prompt emergency referral. Other presenting symptoms include:

- abdominal pain
- pelvic mass due to enlarged uterus
- pyometra: bloody vaginal discharge due to obstruction of the lower uterine cavity which becomes distended with infected secretions
- abnormal glandular cytology or endometrial cells on cervical cytology.

MANAGEMENT

In an emergency situation the primary objective is to provide supportive care and stabilise the situation. This may require transfusion and occasionally an emergency hysterectomy.

In women who are unfit for surgery, bleeding may be brought under control by pelvic radiotherapy. The complications of radiotherapy are shown in Table A2.3.

Vaginal hysterectomy or laparoscopically assisted vaginal hysterectomy can be considered in patients with marked obesity or medical problems placing them at high risk of complications from abdominal surgery. Complications of vaginal hysterectomy include:

- vaginal bleeding: requiring suturing of the vaginal vault
- intra-abdominal bleeding: bleeding from a pedicle requiring laparotomy
- infected vault haematoma: often settle with antibiotics, but may require surgical drainage.

Cervical cancer

It is unusual for cervical cancer to present as an emergency. When it does, bleeding and pain are the most likely presenting symptoms. Rarely, renal failure may be the first presenting symptom although it is usually possible to elicit a history highly suggestive of carcinoma that predates the emergency presentation by several months.

PRESENTATION

Cervical carcinoma often presents early with:

- abnormal vaginal bleeding: postcoital, intermenstrual or postmenopausal. Bleeding be haemorrhagic requiring resuscitation, vaginal packing and rarely, pelvic irradiation or emergency surgery
- vaginal discharge, often bloodstained
- abnormal cervical cytology: detection on subsequent colposcopy.

Late disease presents with:

- malodorous vaginal discharge: infection of tumour bulk with anaerobes
- pelvic pain due to infiltration of the pelvic sidewalls
- referred leg pain due to invasion of the lumbrosacral plexus
- bowel or bladder disturbance: constipation, tenesmus, rectal bleeding, urinary frequency, haematuria or vaginal passage of urine or faeces if a fistula is present
- pelvic mass, in advanced disease
- vesicovaginal and/or rectovaginal fistulae.

INVESTIGATIONS AND STAGING

See Appendix 1 for full details of FIGO staging. A cervical tumour mass is usually visible either macroscopically or colposcopically. If cervical cancer is suspected in an emergency setting, a biopsy can usually be taken without recourse to general anaesthesia. It is not a substitute for formal staging but allows a diagnosis to be made while the patient is stabilised.

Table A2.4 Complications of surgical treatment for cervical cancer

Stage	Treatment	Complications
Ia1	LLETZ Knife cone biopsy	Secondary haemorrhage, due to infection, is treated with bed rest, antibiotics and, rarely, cervical suturing
	Simple hysterectomy	Complications as for laparotomy
Ia2	Knife cone biopsy Wertheim's hysterectomy and lymph node dissection	See Table A2.1 for complications
	Radical trachelectomy	Vaginal procedure with excision of cervix, upper vagina and parametrium (uterine body is left in situ); immediate complications are infection and bleeding
Ib1	Wertheim's hysterectomy and lymph node dissection	See Table A2.1 for complications
Ib2	Preoperative chemoradiation and adjuvant hysterectomy	
IIa	Schauta radical vaginal hysterectomy and lymph node dissection	Involves taking a vaginal cuff, often with enlargement of the vaginal orifice with a Schuchardt's incision (like a large mediolateral episiotomy); decreased operative mortality, c.f. Wertheim's, complications as that for vaginal hysterectomy with increased risk of ureteric damage

TREATMENT

Bleeding can usually be controlled temporarily by vaginal packing with concurrent antibiotics. The latter are required, as secondary infection is one cause of haemorrhage. Blood transfusion may be necessary and even if the bleeding is not profuse, raising the haemoglobin may have treatment effects by enhancing the effect of radiotherapy. Pain should be managed aggressively as part of the initial stabilisation and assessment process. In a minority of situations, haemorrhage is severe and may necessitate additional control measures such as selective embolisation. Once the patient has been stabilised, management follows the pathway for cases presenting in a non-emergency fashion (see Chapters 5 and 12 for full details). Complications of surgical treatment for cervical cancer are given in Table A2.4. Complications of Wertheim hysterectomy and lymph node dissection are as for laparotomy. Haemorrhage occurs at these sites:

- ureteric tunnel
- paracolpos and vaginal edge
- external iliac artery and vein
- obturator fossa
- bifurcation of common iliac artery and vein
- para-aortic lymph nodes (the use of regional anaesthesia reduces small vessel oozing).

Ureteric dysfunction occurs due to:

- damage to the ureteric blood supply
- damage to the ureteric nerve supply
- oedema of the wall of the ureter
- periureteric infection in the retroperitoneal space.

Ureteric stricture and ureterovaginal fistulae develop as late complications and may require surgery. Bladder dysfunction occurs due to:

- damage to sympathetic nerves in uterosacral and cardinal ligaments results in bladder hypertonicity due to parasympathetics
- oedema of bladder neck and muscle
- hypotonicity as a result of overdistension of a hypertonic bladder (catherisation for six to eight days postoperatively is recommended).

Other complications include:

- urinary tract infection
- vesicovaginal fistulae
- pelvic lymphocysts of the pelvic brim or pelvic sidewall can cause pain, obstruction or become infected; they may require surgical drainage
- peripheral leg lymphoedema may develop late and require specialised massage
- nerve damage to the obturator, genitofemoral, femoral, perineal or sciatic nerves
- sexual dysfunction: this is increased if patient receives adjuvant radiotherapy.

Vulval cancer

PRESENTATION

When presenting as an emergency, the usual symptoms will be pain (often resulting in the inability of the patient to sit comfortably), bleeding and urinary retention. Delay in presentation is not unusual in cancer of the vulva, therefore quite advanced disease can present in the emergency situation. As with the other cancers considered in this section, the principles of management remain the same. The patient should be stabilised if necessary, symptom control instituted and then the patient should be assessed and managed as with non-emergency presentation.

In advanced or recurrent disease the groins may be involved with tumour. This raises the possibility of infiltration and rupture of the vessels in the groin. This is a terminal event in vulval cancer. If this occurs, morphine should be administered intravenously to sedate the patient who will be agitated and anxious, packs may be applied to the bleeding area but the excessive haemorrhage inevitably leads to circulatory failure.

The assessment and management of vulval cancer is discussed in Chapter 13.

Further reading

General

MacLean AB, Singer A, Critchley H, editors. *Lower Genital Tract Neoplasia.* London: RCOG; 2003.

NHS Executive. *Guidance On Commissioning Cancer Services. Improving Outcomes in Gynaecological Cancers. The Manual.* London: NHS Executive; 1999.

Chapter 3

Cannistra SA, Niloff JM. Cancer of the uterine cervix. *New Eng J Med* 1996; **334**: 1030–8.

Koutsky L. Epidemiology of genital human papillomavirus infection. *Am J Med* 1997; **102**: 3–8.

Laara E, Day NE, Hakama M. Trends in mortality from cervical cancer in the Nordic countries: association with organised screening programmes. *Lancet* 1987; **i**: 1247–9.

Luesley D, Jordan J, Richart RM. *Intraepithelial Neoplasia of the Lower Genital Tract.* Edinburgh: Churchill Livingstone; 1995.

McIndoe WA, McLean MR, Jones RW, Mullins PR. The invasive potential of carcinoma *in situ* of the cervix. *Obstet Gynecol* 1984; **64**; 451–8.

Wright TC, Richart RM. Role of human papillomavirus in the pathogenesis of genital tract warts and cancer. *Gynecol Oncol* 1990; **37**: 151–64.

Chapter 4

Patnick J, Winder E, editors. *Cervical Screening: A Practical Guide for Health Authorities.* Publication No. 7. Sheffield: NHSCSP; 1997.

NHS Cervical Screening Programme. *Quality Assurance Guidelines for the Cervical Screening Programme: Report of a Working Party convened by the NHS Cervical Screening Programme.* Publication No. 3. Sheffield: NHSCSP; 1996.

Chapter 6

Kadar N. Present and future role of laparoscopic surgery in gynecological oncology. In: Querleu D, Childers JM, Dargent D, editors. *Laparoscopic Surgery in Gynaecological Oncology.* Oxford: Blackwell Science; 1999. p.183–92.

Chapter 7

Dearnaley DP. Principles of radiotherapy. In: Horwich A, editor. *Oncology: A Multidisciplinary Textbook*. London: Chapman & Hall; 1995. p. 117–34.

Hoskin PJ. Radiotherapy in symptom management. In: Doyle D, Hanks GWC, editors. *Oxford Textbook of Palliative Medicine*, 2nd ed. Oxford: Oxford University Press; 1999. p. 267–81.

Chapter 11

NHS Executive. *Guidance on Commissioning Cancer Services. Improving Outcomes in Gynaecological Cancers*. London: Department of Health; 1999.

NHS Executive. *Manuals of Cancer Services Standards*. London: Department of Health; 2000.

NHS Executive. *Health Service Circular: Cancer Waiting Times, Achieving the NHS Cancer Plan Waiting Time Target*. London: Department of Health; 2001.

NHS Executive. *Referral Guidelines for Suspected Cancer*. London: Department of Health; 2000.

Royal College of Obstetricians and Gynaecologists. *Clinical Recommendations for the Management of Vulval Cancer*. London: RCOG; 1999.

Chapter 14

Benedet JL, Saunders BH. Carcinoma *in situ* of the vagina. *Am J Obstet Gynecol* 1984; **148**: 695–700.

Hancock BW, Newlands ES, Berkowitz RS, editors. *Gestational Trophoblastic Disease*. London: Chapman Hall; 1997.

Monaghan JM. Management of vaginal carcinoma. In: Shepherd JH, Monaghan JM, editors. *Clinical Gynaecological Oncology*. London: Blackwell; 1990. p.133–53.

Newlands ES. Clinical management of trophoblastic disease in the United Kingdom. *Curr Obstet Gynecol* 1995; **5**: 19–24.

World Health Organization. *Gestational Trophoblastic Diseases*. Technical Report Series 692. Geneva: WHO; 1983.

Appendix 1

FIGO staging classifications and clinical practice guidelines in the management of gynecologic cancers. *Int J Gynecol Obstet* 2000; **70**: 209–62.

Appendix 2

Byfield JE, Calabro-Jones P, Klisak I, Kulhanian F. Pharmacologic requirements for obtaining sensitization of human tumour cells *in vitro* to combined 5 fluorouracil or ftorafur and X-rays. *Int J Radiat Oncol Biol Phys* 1982; **8**: 1923–32.

Copeland LJ, Gershenson DM, Saul PB, Sneige N, Stringer CA, Edwards CL. Sarcoma botryoides of the female genital tract. *Obstet Gynecol* 1985; **66**: 262–6.

Dancuart F, Delclos L, Taylor WJ, Silva EG. Primary squamous cell carcinoma of the vagina treated by radiotherapy: a failure analysis: the MD Anderson experience 1955–1982. *Int J Radiat Oncol Biol Phys* 1988; **14**: 745–9.

FIGO (International Federation of Obstetrics and Gynecology) Annual report on results of treatment in gynaecological cancer. *Int J Gynecol Cancer* 1989; **28**: 189–90.

Guthrie D, Davy MLJ, Philips PR. Study of 656 patients with "early" ovarian cancer. *Gynecol Oncol* 1984; **17**: 363–9.

Hilgers RD, Malkasian GD, Saule EH. Embryonal rhabdomyosarcoma (botryoid type) of the vagina. A clinicopathologic review. *Am J Obstet Gynecol* 1972; **107**: 484–502.

Homesley HD, Bundy BN, Sedlis A, Adcock L. Radiation therapy versus node resection for carcinoma of the vulva with positive groin nodes. *Obstet Gynecol* 1986; **68**: 733–40.

Keys HM, Bundy BN, Stehman FB, Muderspach LI, Chafe WE, Suggs CL 3rd, *et al*. Cisplatin, radiation and adjuvant hysterectomy compared with radiation and adjuvant hysterectomy for bulky Stage Ib cervical carcinoma. *N Engl J Med* 1999; **340**: 1154–61.

Kirkbride P, Fyles A, Rawlings GA, Manchul L, Levin W, Murphy KJ, *et al*. Carcinoma of the vagina – experience at the Princess Margaret Hospital (1974–1989). *Gynecol Oncol* 1995; **56**: 435–43.

Knocke TH, Kucera H, Dotfler D, Pokrajac B, Potter R. Results of post-operative radiotherapy in the treatment of sarcoma of the corpus uteri. *Cancer* 1998; **83**: 1972–9.

Janicke F, Holscher M, Kuhn W, von Hugo R, Pache L, Siewert JR, *et al*. Radical surgical procedure improves survival time in patients with recurrent ovarian cancer. *Cancer* 1992; **70**: 2129–36.

Nanavati PJ, Fanning J, Hilgers RD, Hallstrom J, Crawford D. High-dose-rate brachytherapy in primary stage I and II vaginal cancer. *Gynecol Oncol* 1993; **51**: 67–71.

Morris M, Eifel PJ, Lu J, Grigsby PW, Levenback C, Stevens RE, *et al*. Pelvic radiation with concurrent chemotherapy compared with pelvic and para-aortic radiation for high-risk cervical cancer. *N Engl J Med* 1999; **340**: 1137–43.

Peters WA 3rd, Liu PY, Barrett RJ 2nd, Stock RJ, Monk BJ, Berek JS, *et al*. Concurrent chemotherapy and pelvic radiation therapy compared with pelvic radiation therapy alone as adjuvant therapy after radical surgery in high-risk early-stage cancer of the cervix. *J Clin Oncol* 2000; **18**: 1606–13.

Rose PG, Bundy BN, Watkins EB, Thigpen JT, Deppe G, Maiman MA, *et al*. Concurrent cisplatin-based radiotherapy and for locally advanced cervical cancer. *N Eng J Med* 1999; **340**: 1144–53 (erratum in *N Engl J Med* 1999; **341**: 708).

Thomas G, Dembo A, DePetrillo A, Pringle J, Ackerman I, Bryson P, *et al*. Concurrent radiation and chemotherapy in vulvar carcinoma. *Gynecol Oncol* 1989; **34**: 263–7.

van der Burg ME, van Lent M, Buyse M, Kobierska A, Colombo N, Favalli G, *et al*. The effect of debulking surgery after induction chemotherapy on the prognosis in advanced epithelial ovarian cancer. *N Eng J Med* 1995; **332**: 629–34.

Whitney CW, Sause W, Bundy BN, Malfetano JH, Hannigan EV, Fowler WC Jr, *et al*. Randomized comparison of fluorouracil plus cisplatin versus hydroxyurea as an adjunct to radiation therapy in stage IIB-IVA carcinoma of the cervix with negative para-aortic nodes: a Gynecologic Oncology Group and Southwest Oncology Group study. *J Clin Oncol* 1999; **17**: 1339–48.

Useful websites

These websites can be accessed free of charge and have image libraries. They can also provide useful links.

CHAPTER 1

Cancer Research Campaign [www.crc.org.uk]

CHAPTER 2

www.digitalpathology.com

www.pathweb.uchc.edu

www.medlib.med.utah.edu

www.cytopathnet.org

www.pathology.ks.se

CHAPTER 3

NHS Cervical Screening Programme [www.cancerscreening.nhs.uk/cervical/index.html].
All of the NHSCSP publications can be accessed from this site and many can be downloaded as PDF files.

National Institute of Clinical Excellence [www.nice.org.uk].

British Society for Colposcopy and Cervical Pathology [www.bsccp.org.uk].
This is the website of the BSCCP. Some of the pages are secure and can only be accessed by members or trainees. However, there are pages designed to give general information on preinvasive disease, including images and video clips, and there are many links to similar sites.

American Society for Colposcopy and Cervical Pathology [www.asccp.org].
This is the American society's website and is quite sophisticated in design. You can take part in the colposcopy challenge based on images and case scenarios.

Royal College of Obstetricians and Gynaecologists [www.rcog.org.uk]
The RCOG site contains the report of a working party on Recommendation for Service Provision and Standards in Colposcopy.

Oncolink [http://cancer.med.upenn.edu]
This is a huge site with a wealth of information on all cancers. It is well designed and includes online MS Powerpoint lectures. These ideally need a fast modem.

Index

PUBLISHED TITLES IN THE MRCOG & BEYOND SERIES

The books in this series are an invaluable aid, not only for candidates preparing to sit the MRCOG examination but also for those in clinical practice, midwives and, indeed, any health professional who comes into contact with women.

All titles in this series are available from the RCOG Bookshop

Tel: +44 (0) 20 7772 6275;
fax: +44 (0) 20 7724 5991;
email: bookshop@rcog.org.uk
Buy online at www.rcogbookshop.com

Reproductive Endocrinology for the MRCOG and Beyond

Edited by Adam Balen

To understand endocrinology is to understand the key processes that affect normal reproductive function. A knowledge of normal endocrinology and the pathophysiology of endocrine disorders is important when dealing with disorders of reproduction. *Reproductive Endocrinology for the MRCOG and Beyond* aims to provide a comprehensive background for all gynaecologists.

Contents: Preface; Abbreviations; Sexual differentiation: intersex disorders; Adrenal disorders; Normal puberty and adolescence; Abnormal puberty; The menstrual cycle; Disorders of menstruation; Amenorrhoea; Polycystic ovary syndrome; Health consequences of polycystic ovary syndrome; Anovulatory infertility and ovulation induction; Lactation and lactational amenorrhoea; Hyperprolactinaemia; Thyroid disease; Diabetes; Lipid metabolism and lipoprotein transport; Premature ovarian failure; Calcium metabolism and its disorders; Appendix1: Endocrine normal ranges; Further reading; Index.

1-900364-83-2	197 pages	Published 2003

Fetal Medicine for the MRCOG and Beyond

Alan Cameron, Lena Macara, Janet Brennand, Peter Milton

A working knowledge of fetal medicine is essential for both aspiring specialists in obstetrics and gynaecology and established practitioners. This book comprehensively covers the whole field, with contributions relating not only to diagnostic techniques but also, most importantly, to the management of fetal abnormality following diagnosis. It is an important addition to the literature relating to this extremely exciting and rapidly advancing field of obstetric practice.

Contents: Preface; Abbreviations; Screening for chromosomal abnormalities; Prenatal diagnostic techniques; The routine anomaly scan; Fetal structural abnormalities; Prenatal diagnosis and management of non-immune hydrops fetalis; Termination of pregnancy for fetal abnormality; Intrauterine growth restriction; Twin pregnancy; Index.

1-900364-74-3	152 pages	Published 2003

Intrapartum Care for the MRCOG and Beyond

Thomas F Baskett and Sabatnam Arulkumaran

This book provides a balanced but pragmatic guide to clinical intrapartum care. It is an invaluable aid, not only for candidates preparing to sit the MRCOG examination but also for those in clinical practice, midwives and, indeed, any health professional who comes into contact with mothers.

Contents: Preface; Abbreviations; Introduction; First stage of labour; second stage of labour; Fetal surveillance in labour; Third stage of labour; Induction of labour; Preterm labour and prelabour rupture of membranes; Assisted vaginal delivery; Breech vaginal delivery; Twin and triplet delivery; Caesarean section; Vaginal birth after caesarean section; Uterine rupture and emergency hysterectomy; Shoulder dystocia; Cord prolapse; Antepartum haemorrhage; Postpartum haemorrhage; Amniotic fluid embolism; Severe pre-eclampsia and eclampsia; Neonatal resuscitation by John McIntyre; Perinatal loss by Carolyn Basak; Further reading; Index.

1-900364-73-5	224 pages	Published 2002

Menopause for the MRCOG and Beyond

Margaret Rees

The management of the menopause and hormone replacement therapy has become an increasingly important subject for the MRCOG examinations in recent years. This review provides the MRCOG trainee with an excellent insight and with more than enough current facts and figures, but it will also be extremely useful for anyone else wishing to be up-to-date in this increasingly important area.

Contents: Preface; Introduction, definitions and physiology; Consequences of ovarian failure; Investigations; Benefits of HRT; Risks of HRT; HRT: preparations, prescribing, treatment duration and management of adverse effects; Specific pre-existing medical conditions and HRT; Monitoring HRT; Non-hormone replacement therapy and osteoporosis; Complementary and alternative therapies; Index.

1-900364-45-X	98 pages	Published 2002

Paediatric and Adolescent Gynaecology for the MRCOG and Beyond

Anne Garden and Joanne Topping

A broad knowledge of caring for children and adolescents with gynaecological disorders is essential for everyone in clinical practice. All clinicians, at some point in their careers, will be required to deal with young people who present with symptoms that could possibly be due to gynaecological pathology. This book covers the whole range of developments in the field of paediatric and adolescent gynaecology, ranging from conditions specific to childhood to contraception, female genital mutilation and gynaecological malignancies. The subject is dealt with in a sensitive and understanding manner and is clearly written by authors with a worldwide reputation in the field. It is an invaluable aid, not only for candidates preparing to sit the MRCOG examination but also for those in clinical practice, midwives and, indeed, any health professional who comes into contact with young people.

Contents: Preface; Pubertal growth and development; Indeterminate genitalia; Gynaecological problems in childhood; Endocrine disorders; Child sexual abuse; Amenorrhoea; Menstrual problems in teenagers; Contraception; Female genital mutilation; Gynaecological tumours; Index.

1-900364-42-5	96 pages	Published 2001

Antenatal Disorders for the MRCOG and Beyond

Andrew Thompson and Ian Greer

Patterns and provision of antenatal care have changed enormously in recent years in response to the opinions of consumers, providers, professional associations and government reports. During pregnancy, most women remain well and require little formal medical input. For them, pregnancy is a physiological process. However, some women develop complications with significant morbidity or mortality for their baby and, occasionally, for themselves. Providers of antenatal care must be able to distinguish between these two groups of women and arrange with them an appropriate and personalised plan of care.

This volume encompasses all aspects of identifying and caring for those women who develop disorders during their pregnancies.

Contents: Preface; Antenatal care and risk assessment; Assessment of fetal growth and well-being; Antepartum haemorrhage; Multiple pregnancy; Preterm labour; Hypertensive disorders of pregnancy; Common medical disorders in pregnancy; Rhesus disease; Recommended reading; Index.

1-900364-36-0	208 pages	Published 2000

Management of Infertility for the MRCOG and Beyond

Allan Templeton, P Ashok, S Bhattacharya, R Gazvani, M Hamilton, S MacMillan & A Shetty

Every MRCOG candidate must have a broad knowledge of infertility management. Infertility affects one in seven couples in the Western world and this figure may rise as more women are delaying parenthood. It is a major cause of psychological and marital stress and, hence, deserves to be managed as a disease entity along with more traditionally recognised diseases

This volume has been written jointly by members of one of the most prestigious infertility clinics in the UK (Aberdeen Maternity Hospital) and provides information on all aspects of infertility, both male and female.

Contents: Preface; The management of infertility; The initial assessment of the infertile couple; Male factor infertility; Disorders of ovulation; Tubal-factor infertility; Infertility and endometriosis; Unexplained infertility; Assisted conception techniques; Glossary; Recommended reading; Index.

1-900364-29-8	131 pages	Published 2000

Gynaecological and Obstetric Pathology for the MRCOG

Harold Fox and Hilary Buckley

This succinct and copiously illustrated volume covers pathological conditions of the vulva, vagina, uterus, fallopian tube and ovary, in addition to abnormalities related to pregnancy, and cervical cytology. Gynaecological and Obstetric Pathology is an invaluable revision text for candidates preparing for the Part 1 and Part 2 MRCOG Examination, and is in addition a readily accessible, concise and up-to-date reference text for practising clinicians.

Contents: Preface; The vulva; The vagina; The cervix; The endometrium; The myometrium; The fallopian tube; The ovary; Abnormalities related to pregnancy; Cervical cytology, *by Dulcie V Coleman*; Suggested references for further reading; Index.

0-902331-84-1	184 pages	Published 1998